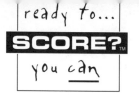

ready to...

SCORE?™

you can

SO-BIM-235

ScoreCards™ for
Vascular Technology

A Q&A Flashcard Study System for Vascular Technology

DAVIES
PUBLISHING

By Cindy Owen, RDMS, RVT
D. E. Strandness, Jr., MD, Series Editor

Library of Congress Cataloging-in-Publication Data

Owen, Cindy.

ScoreCards for vascular technology : a Q & A flashcard study system for vascular technology / by Cindy Owen,
D. E. Strandness, Jr.

p.; cm.

ISBN 0-941022-48-X

1. Blood-vessels–Diseases–Ultrasonic imaging–Examinations, questions, etc.

[DNLM: 1. Vascular Diseases–ultrasonography–Examination Questions. WG 18.2 O97s 2000] I. Title: Vascular
technology. II. Strandness, D. E. (Donald Eugene), 1928–. III. Title.

RC691.6.U47 O94 2000

616.1'307543'076–dc21

00-060161

Davies Publishing, Inc.

32 South Raymond Avenue
Pasadena, California 91105-1935
website www.daviespublishing.com/telephone 626-792-3046

Cover and text design by Bill Murawski / Prepress production by The Left Coast Group, Inc.
Printed and bound in the United States of America

ISBN 0-941022-48-X

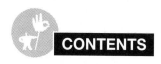

CONTENTS

III

The *ScoreCards* study system follows the ARDMS outline for the Vascular Technology (VT) examination. The *ScoreCards* contents are therefore the same as the ARDMS outline. As in the ARDMS outline, the numbers in parentheses indicate the approximate percentage of the exam that a particular subject will represent. On the question side of each page of the *ScoreCards*, at the bottom, there is a key indicating its place within this outline, as well as the relative importance of the topic. So you always know where you are and how you are doing.

In addition to covering the ARDMS exam content outline, *ScoreCards for Vascular Technology* also contains an image gallery of challenging case-based problems <u>and</u> bonus coverage of the *Fluid Dynamics* section of the Vascular Physical Principles and Instrumentation (VPI) examination—the other exam that a registry candidate must pass to earn the RVT credential. You get not only complete and accurate coverage of the VT exam, but also a free preview of both the VPI examination (part 3, Physiology and Fluid Dynamics) and *ScoreCards for Vascular Physics*, the Step 3 study system for that exam.

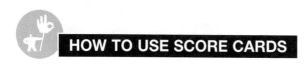

HOW TO USE SCORE CARDS

As part of our 1-2-3 Step Ultrasound Education and Test Preparation program, *ScoreCards for Vascular Technology* systematically prepares you to pass the Vascular Technology exam for the RVT credential. It also helps you to master the facts, problem-solving skills, and habits of mind that form the foundation of success not only on your registry exams but also in your career as an ultrasound professional. And they're fun. Here are some tips for maximizing their value:

Take it with you. The pocket-sized *ScoreCards* study system is designed to be portable. Use it on breaks or between patients. You can review a dozen question/answer items in five minutes.

Study, test yourself, review. As you study vascular technology, *ScoreCards* drills you on key facts and figures, it tests your knowledge of those facts in practical situations, and it provides clear explanations and references for further study. Each Q&A card is keyed to the ARDMS exam content outline so that you always know where you are, how you are doing, and how important the topic is to your overall success on the exam.

Triangulate on your target. By itself, the *ScoreCards* study system is a powerful, convenient, and fun way of learning and testing yourself. It is especially effective when used with *Vascular Technology: An Illustrated Review* [Step 1: review text] and *Vascular Technology Review* [Step 2: mock examination]. Just as each ScoreCard tells you which exam topic it covers, it also indicates exactly where in the Step 1 text you can find further information about the subject. So do the

Davies mock examinations. This integrated, systematic strategy triangulates on your target—exam and career success!

Shuffle it! After using the flipcard format for a while, consider removing the spiral wire binding and mixing up the cards to vary the order in which they challenge you.

Earn CME credit. The *ScoreCards* study system is an SDMS-approved CME activity that can help you earn the 12 clock hours required to take an ARDMS exam or to meet the CME requirements necessary to maintain your registry status once you pass your exams. Use the application that follows the last question in this book.

Check our website. News about your exams, continuing medical education, diagnostic testing, catalogs of additional references and resources, and online help are just a click away. Visit us at daviespublishing.com or readytoscore.com.

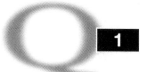

Q 1

In this illustration of the aortic arch, name the vessels labeled A–E.

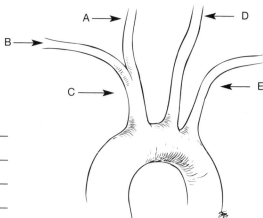

a. _____

b. _____

c. _____

d. _____

e. _____

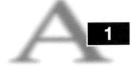

A. Right common carotid artery.

B. Right subclavian artery

C. Innominate artery.

D. Left common carotid artery.

E. Left subclavian artery.

This classic pattern of the aortic arch is seen in approximately 70% of individuals. The first of these branches is the innominate or brachiocephalic trunk, which usually courses 3–4 cm before dividing into the right common carotid and subclavian arteries. The second branch is the left common carotid artery. The last branch of the aortic arch is the left subclavian artery.

▶ Kadir S: Regional anatomy of the thoracic aorta. In *Atlas of Normal and Variant Angiographic Anatomy.* Philadelphia, Saunders, 1991, pp 19–54.

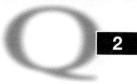

2

The most common anatomic variant of the aortic arch is:

a.   a common origin of the innominate and left common carotid arteries

b.   origin of the left vertebral from the aortic arch

c.   origin of the right subclavian from the aortic arch

d.   origin of the right common carotid from the aortic arch

I–IV. Vascular Anatomy, Physiology, and Hemodynamics / Cerebrovascular and Peripheral Arterial (1–5%)

A **2**

A. A common origin of the innominate and left common carotid arteries.

A common origin of the innominate and left common carotid arteries is by far the most common variant anatomy of the aortic arch, occurring in approximately 22% of individuals.

▶ Kadir S: Regional anatomy of the thoracic aorta. In *Atlas of Normal and Variant Angiographic Anatomy.* Philadelphia, Saunders, 1991, pp 19–54.

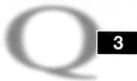

3

The subclavian artery becomes known as what artery after crossing the lateral margin of the first rib?

a. brachiocephalic artery

b. axillary artery

c. brachial artery

d. vertebral artery

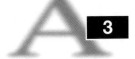

3

B. Axillary artery.

The subclavian artery continues as the axillary artery after it passes the lateral margin of the first rib. The axillary artery in turn becomes the brachial artery.

▶ Rumwell C, McPharlin M: *Vascular Technology: An Illustrated Review,* 2nd edition. Pasadena, Davies Publishing, 2000, p 2.

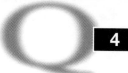

4

The common hepatic, splenic, and left gastric arteries are branches arising from what abdominal artery?

a. superior mesenteric artery

b. proper hepatic artery

c. inferior mesenteric artery

d. celiac trunk

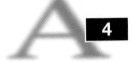

D. Celiac trunk.

The celiac is the first major branch of the abdominal aorta. It divides into the common hepatic, splenic and left gastric arteries.

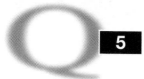

Q **5**

What is the most common anatomic variation of the renal arteries?

a. retroaortic renal artery

b. multiple renal arteries

c. congenital absence of one main renal artery

d. anterocaval course of right renal artery

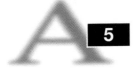

5

B. Multiple renal arteries.

The presence of multiple renal arteries is the most common anatomic variant of the renal arteries, occurring in up to 30% of individuals. Multiple renal arteries occur with equal frequency on both sides and may occur unilaterally or bilaterally. They most commonly originate from the abdominal aorta or common iliac arteries but may arise from the superior and inferior mesenteric, median sacral, intercostal, lumbar, adrenal, inferior French, right hepatic, or right colic arteries. These anomalous origins of the renal arteries are commonly seen in individuals with ectopic or horseshoe kidneys.

▶ Rumwell C, McPharlin M: *Vascular Technology: An Illustrated Review,* 2nd edition. Pasadena, Davies Publishing, 2000, pp 6–7.

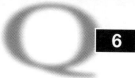

6

The tiny intrarenal branches that arise at right angles from the interlobar arteries and course above the renal pyramids are the:

a. arcuate arteries

b. interlobular arteries

c. capsular arteries

d. segmental arteries

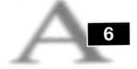

A. Arcuate arteries.

The main renal artery divides at the hilum of the kidney into segmental renal arteries. These in turn give rise to the interlobar arteries, which course alongside the renal pyramids. The arcuate arteries arise at right angles from the interlobar arteries and course on top of the renal pyramids. Within the renal cortex, the arcuate arteries give rise to the radially oriented interlobular arteries.

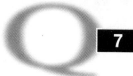

7

At the inguinal ligament, the external iliac artery becomes what peripheral artery?

a. internal iliac artery
b. profunda femoral artery
c. common femoral artery
d. superficial femoral artery

A 7

C. Common femoral artery.

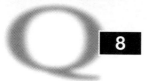

8

The dorsalis pedis is a continuation of which of the following arteries?

a. anterior tibial artery
b. posterior tibial artery
c. peroneal artery
d. popliteal artery

A 8

A. Anterior tibial artery.

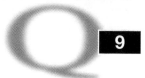

9

The small intestine, right colon, and transverse colon are supplied by the:

a. gastroduodenal artery
b. superior mesenteric artery
c. inferior mesenteric artery
d. left gastric artery

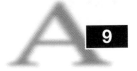

9

B. Superior mesenteric artery.

The superior mesenteric artery (SMA) is the second major branch of the abdominal aorta. It arises approximately 1 cm below the origin of the celiac trunk. Major branches of the SMA include the inferior pancreaticoduodenal artery, jejunal and ileal branches, ileocolic artery, right colic artery, and the middle colic artery. The inferior mesenteric artery (IMA) feeds the left third of the transverse colon, the sigmoid colon, and part of the rectum. It is usually much smaller than the SMA. It arises on the left ventral aspect of the abdominal aorta a few centimeters before the aortic bifurcation. Its major branches include the left colic artery, sigmoid branches, and superior rectal artery.

▶ Rumwell C, McPharlin M: *Vascular Technology: An Illustrated Review,* 2nd edition. Pasadena, Davies Publishing, 2000, pp 6–7.

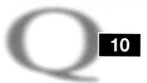

10

The largest branch of the celiac trunk is the:

a. splenic artery

b. hepatic artery

c. left gastric artery

d. gastroduodenal artery

A `10`

A. Splenic artery.

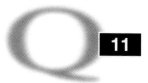

11

The hypogastric artery is another name for the:

a. gastroduodenal artery

b. hepatic artery

c. external iliac artery

d. internal iliac artery

DAVIES
Registry Reviews & Study Aids

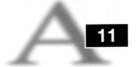

D. Internal iliac artery.

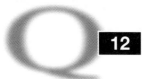

12

Which of the following vessels courses along the medial aspect of the psoas muscle?

a. internal iliac artery
b. external iliac artery
c. femoral artery
d. inferior mesenteric artery

A `12`

B. External iliac artery.

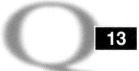

13

The first branch of the external carotid artery is usually the:

a. facial artery
b. superficial temporal artery
c. internal maxillary artery
d. superior thyroid artery

A 13

D. Superior thyroid artery.

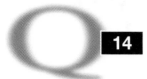

Q **14**

The vertebral artery enters the transverse foramina of the cervical spine at what level?

a. C1

b. C7

c. C6

d. C2

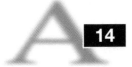

C. C6.

▶ Kadir S: Regional anatomy of the thoracic aorta. In *Atlas of Normal and Variant Angiographic Anatomy*. Philadelphia, Saunders, 1991, pp 19–54.

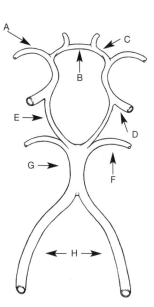

In this illustration of the circle of Willis, name the vessels that are labeled.

a. _____

b. _____

c. _____

d. _____

e. _____

f. _____

g. _____

h. _____

I–IV. Vascular Anatomy, Physiology, and Hemodynamics / Cerebrovascular (1–5%)

A 15

A. Middle cerebral artery.

B. Anterior communicating artery.

C. Anterior cerebral artery.

D. Internal carotid artery.

E. Posterior communicating artery.

F. Posterior cerebral artery.

G. Basilar artery.

H. Vertebral artery.

▶ Rumwell C, McPharlin M: *Vascular Technology: An Illustrated Review,* 2nd edition. Pasadena, Davies Publishing, 2000, pp 123–126.

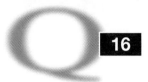

16

The three major branches of the ophthalmic artery are:

a. frontal, supraorbital, and nasal arteries
b. superficial temporal, angular, and facial arteries
c. orbital, facial, and nasal arteries
d. frontal, nasal, and lacrimal arteries

A **16**

A. Frontal, supraorbital, nasal.

▶ Uflacker R: *Atlas of Vascular Anatomy—An Angiographic Approach*. Baltimore, Williams and Wilkins, 1997.

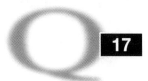

Q 17

The basilar artery divides into which of the following arteries?

a. posterior communicating arteries
b. posterior cerebral arteries
c. vertebral arteries
d. posterior inferior cerebellar arteries

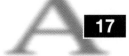

A 17

B. Posterior cerebral arteries.

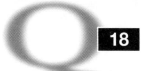

18

The external carotid artery provides an anastomotic link to the internal carotid artery through the orbit via which of the following vessels?

a. superficial temporal artery
b. superior thyroid artery
c. internal maxillary artery
d. posterior communicating artery

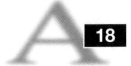

A. Superficial temporal artery.

The external carotid artery (ECA) can supply the internal carotid artery (ICA) when needed through the periorbital circulation. The three main arteries arising from the ophthalmic artery (supraorbital, frontal, and nasal) have anastomotic links with ECA branches. These connections can provide blood flow to the intracranial circulation in the case of ICA occlusion via retrograde flow through the ophthalmic artery. The supraorbital and frontal arteries connect to the ECA through the superficial temporal artery. The nasal artery becomes the angular artery as it descends along the lateral border of the nose and connects to the ECA via the facial artery.

▶ Rumwell C, McPharlin M: *Vascular Technology: An Illustrated Review,* 2nd edition. Pasadena, Davies Publishing, 2000, pp 121–126.
▶ Ridgway DP: *Introduction to Vascular Scanning: A Guide for the Complete Beginner,* 2nd edition. Pasadena, Davies Publishing, 1999, pp 39–43.

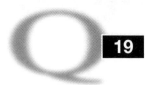

19

All of the following arise from the intracranial internal carotid artery **EXCEPT:**

a. middle cerebral artery
b. anterior cerebral artery
c. ascending pharyngeal
d. posterior communicating artery

A 19

C. Ascending pharyngeal.

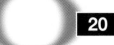

20

The ophthalmic artery is a branch of the:

a. anterior communicating artery

b. anterior cerebral artery

c. external carotid artery

d. internal carotid artery

A 20

D. Internal carotid artery.

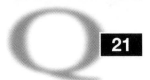

21

In the case of internal carotid artery occlusion, all of the following are potential collateral pathways to perfuse the ipsilateral cerebral hemisphere **EXCEPT**:

a. contralateral internal carotid artery through reversed flow in the ipsilateral anterior cerebral artery

b. vertebrobasilar system through the posterior communicating artery

c. ipsilateral external carotid artery through the orbit to the ophthalmic artery

d. contralateral subclavian artery to the internal mammary artery

A 21

D. Contralateral subclavian artery to the internal mammary artery.

This is NOT a collateral pathway to the cerebral hemisphere. All other answers are potential collateral pathways.

Q 22

Which branch of the external carotid artery provides a collateral pathway to the vertebral artery?

a. lingual artery

b. occipital artery

c. facial artery

d. superficial temporal artery

A 22

B. Occipital.

▶ Rumwell C, McPharlin M: *Vascular Technology: An Illustrated Review,* 2nd edition. Pasadena, Davies Publishing, 2000.
▶ Ridgway DP: *Introduction to Vascular Scanning: A Guide for the Complete Beginner,* 2nd edition. Pasadena, Davies Publishing, 1999, pp 39–43.

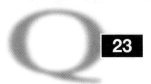

23

In the case of vertebral artery occlusion, which vessel is likely to be enlarged?

a. ipsilateral external carotid artery

b. contralateral internal mammary artery

c. contralateral vertebral artery

d. ipsilateral subclavian artery

A **23**

C. Contralateral vertebral.

In the case of vertebral artery occlusion, compensatory enlargement of the contralateral vertebral is quite common.

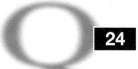

Q 24

A 48-year-old male presents with retrograde flow in the left vertebral artery. This is most likely related to occlusion of the:

a. left subclavian artery
b. right vertebral artery
c. right subclavian artery
d. innominate artery

A **24**

A. Left subclavian artery.

In the case of proximal left subclavian artery occlusion, the left vertebral artery flow will reverse to provide blood flow to the left arm. This condition is termed subclavian steal. Although it occurs more commonly on the left side, it can be present on either side of the body.

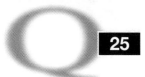

25

What is the most common anomaly of the circle of Willis?

a. absence of one of the middle cerebral arteries
b. duplication of the posterior communicating arteries
c. hypoplasia of the proximal segment of one of the anterior cerebral arteries
d. absence or hypoplasia of one or both of the communicating arteries

A `25`

D. Absence or hypoplasia of one or both of the communicating arteries.

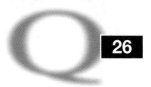

26

Which of the following is **NOT** a branch of the subclavian artery?

a. vertebral artery
b. thyrocervical trunk
c. internal mammary artery
d. brachial artery

A 26

D. Brachial artery.

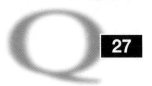

Q 27

Differentiation of the cervical internal carotid artery from the external carotid artery can be accomplished by all of the following **EXCEPT:**

a. The external carotid artery gives off multiple branches in the neck.

b. The internal carotid artery is usually located anteromedial to the external carotid artery.

c. There are normally no branches of the internal carotid artery in the neck.

d. A bulbous area is seen at the origin of the internal carotid artery.

A 27

B. This statement—"the internal carotid artery is usually located anteromedial to the external carotid artery"—is NOT true.

The internal carotid artery is usually located lateral and posterior to the external carotid artery.

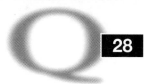

28

Which of the following vessels joins the brachial veins to form the axillary vein?

a. subclavian vein

b. innominate vein

c. cephalic vein

d. basilic vein

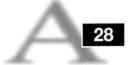

28

D. Basilic vein.

The basilic vein is a superficial vein of the upper extremity that joins with the brachial veins to form the axillary vein. It begins on the ulnar side of the forearm and crosses ventrally at the antecubital region. The basilic vein lies medial to the brachial artery in the upper arm.

▶ Rumwell C, McPharlin M: *Vascular Technology: An Illustrated Review,* 2nd edition. Pasadena, Davies Publishing, 2000, pp 174, 205.

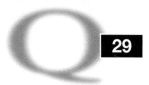

29

Which vein in the antecubital fossa connects the cephalic and basilic veins?

a. axillary vein
b. median cubital vein
c. cephalic vein
d. basilic vein

I-IV. Vascular Anatomy, Physiology, and Hemodynamics / Venous (1–5%)

A 29

B. Median cubital vein.

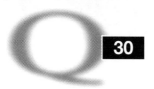

30

All of the following are deep veins of the upper extremity **EXCEPT:**

a. brachial vein

b. cephalic vein

c. axillary vein

d. radial vein

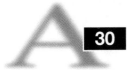

B. Cephalic vein.

The deep veins of the upper extremity include the deep palmar venous arch, radial veins, ulnar veins and interosseous veins of the forearm, brachial veins, and axillary vein. The deep veins accompany the same named arteries and are usually paired. The cephalic, basilic, and median cubital veins are superficial veins. They do not accompany an artery and are not paired.

▶ Rumwell C, McPharlin M: *Vascular Technology: An Illustrated Review,* 2nd edition. Pasadena, Davies Publishing, 2000, pp 174, 205, 242.

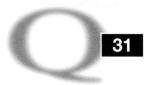

31

The brachiocephalic vein is found:

a. only on the right side of the neck
b. only on the left side of the neck
c. on both the right and left sides of the neck
d. there is no such vein

A `31`

C. On both sides of the neck.

The venous anatomy of the neck varies from the arterial anatomy in that the brachiocephalic *vein* occurs bilaterally, whereas the brachiocephalic (innominate) *artery* is found only on the right side. The brachiocephalic vein is formed by the junction of the subclavian and internal jugular veins.

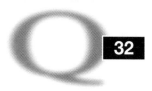

32

The longest vein in the body is the:

a. greater saphenous vein
b. basilic vein
c. femoral vein
d. posterior tibial vein

A **32**

A. Greater saphenous vein.

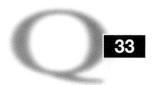

33

Which of the following is **NOT** true regarding perforating veins?

a. They have one valve each.

b. They direct blood from the deep system into the superficial system.

c. They are more numerous in the calf than in the thigh.

d. They are known as varicose veins when they are tortuous and dilated due to incompetent valves.

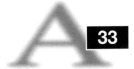 **33**

B. They direct blood from the deep system into the superficial system.

Perforating veins do NOT direct blood from the deep system into the superficial system. They direct blood flow from the superficial system (greater and lesser saphenous veins) into the deep system. All of the other statements are true.

▶ Rumwell C, McPharlin M: *Vascular Technology: An Illustrated Review,* 2nd edition. Pasadena, Davies Publishing, 2000, pp 172–173, 176, 179–180, 184.

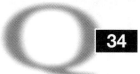

34

The portal vein is formed by the junction of which of the following veins?

a. splenic and superior mesenteric veins

b. superior mesenteric and left gastric veins

c. inferior mesenteric and splenic veins

d. umbilical and splenic veins

A 34

A. Splenic and superior mesenteric veins.

35

What vein normally courses between the superior mesenteric artery and the abdominal aorta?

a.   portal vein

b.   superior mesenteric vein

c.   left renal vein

d.   inferior mesenteric vein

A `35`

C. Left renal vein.

The normal course of the left renal vein is between the abdominal aorta and the superior mesenteric artery. Rarely, it may course behind the abdominal aorta as a retroaortic left renal vein, or it may form a ring around the aorta as a circumaortic left renal vein.

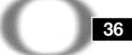

36

Which statement is **NOT** true regarding the soleal veins?

a. They empty into the posterior tibial or peroneal veins.
b. They are found deep in the calf muscle.
c. They connect with the superficial venous system.
d. They do not contain valves.

A 36

C. This statement—"they connect with the superficial venous system"—is NOT true. The soleal veins DO NOT connect with the superficial venous system of the leg.

▶ Rumwell C, McPharlin M: *Vascular Technology: An Illustrated Review,* 2nd edition. Pasadena, Davies Publishing, 2000, pp 172, 237.

Q **37**

Boyd's vein is a perforating vein that connects the gastrocnemius veins to the:

a. anterior tibial veins
b. posterior tibial veins
c. peroneal veins
d. popliteal veins

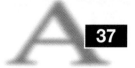

37

B. Posterior tibial veins.

In the leg, there are 16 constant perforating veins. Eight of these drain into the posterior tibial veins. These are known as *Boyd's veins* and *Cockett's veins.* There are 4 perforating veins that drain into the peroneal veins and 4 that drain into the soleal and genicular veins. In the thigh, there are 2 constant perforating veins. These are known as *Dodd's group* or the *perforating veins of Hunter.*

▶ Uflacker R: *Atlas of Vascular Anatomy—An Angiographic Approach.* Baltimore, Williams and Wilkins, 1997.

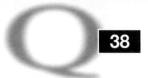

38

The splenic vein drains into which of the following veins?

a. inferior vena cava
b. portal vein
c. hepatic vein
d. superior mesenteric vein

I–IV. Vascular Anatomy, Physiology, and Hemodynamics / Venous / Microscopic Anatomy (1–5%)

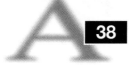

B. Portal vein.

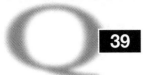

39

The hepatic veins drain into the:

a. portal veins
b. hepatic arteries
c. superior mesenteric vein
d. inferior vena cava

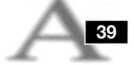

39

D. Inferior vena cava.

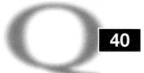

40

Regarding the inferior vena cava, all of the statements below are true **EXCEPT:**

a.   The inferior vena cava drains into the left atrium of the heart.

b.   The inferior vena cava is formed by the confluence of the common iliac veins.

c.   The inferior vena cava has no valves below the level of its insertion into the heart.

d.   The inferior vena cava courses to the right of the abdominal aorta.

I–IV. Vascular Anatomy, Physiology, and Hemodynamics / Venous / Microscopic Anatomy (1–5%)

A **40**

A. This statement—"the IVC drains into the left atrium of the heart"—is NOT true.
The IVC drains into the RIGHT atrium of the heart.

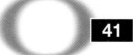

41

The outermost layer of the arterial wall is the:

a. intima

b. media

c. adventitia

d. fascia

I–IV. Vascular Anatomy, Physiology, and Hemodynamics / Peripheral Arterial / Microscopic Anatomy (1–5%)

A 41

C. Adventitia.

The three layers of the arterial wall from the outermost to the innermost are the adventitia, media, and intima.

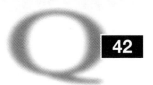

42

The major function of the vasa vasorum is to:

a. regulate vasodilatation of the arterioles

b. provide nourishment to the tunica adventitia

c. provide the major communication in arteriovenous fistulas

d. provide autoregulation of blood flow to the brain

A **42**

B. Provide nourishment to the tunica adventitia.

▶ Rumwell C, McPharlin M: *Vascular Technology: An Illustrated Review,* 2nd edition. Pasadena, Davies Publishing, 2000, pp 126, 175.
▶ Belanger AC: *Vascular Anatomy and Physiology.* Pasadena, Davies Publishing, 1999, p 25.

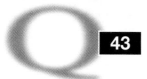

43

What is the function of the semilunar valves of the veins?

a. direct the flow of blood away from the heart
b. provide nourishment to the tunica intima
c. prevent communication between arteries and veins
d. maintain unidirectional flow within the venous system

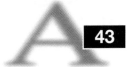

43

D. Maintain unidirectional flow within the venous system.

The semilunar valves of the veins are designed to direct the flow of blood back toward the heart by closing during retrograde flow.

▶ Rumwell C, McPharlin M: *Vascular Technology: An Illustrated Review,* 2nd edition. Pasadena, Davies Publishing, 2000, p 175–180.

▶ Belanger AC: *Vascular Anatomy and Physiology.* Pasadena, Davies Publishing, 1999, p 177–179.

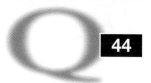

44

Which of the following veins has the greatest number of valves?

a. common femoral vein

b. popliteal vein

c. femoral vein

d. greater saphenous vein

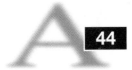

D. Greater saphenous vein (GSV).

The GSV typically has 10–12 valves throughout its length. Other veins are listed below:
* lesser saphenous, 6–12
* soleal sinuses, none
* perforators, 1 valve each
* infrapopliteal (deep veins), 9–12 valves each
* popliteal and femoral, 1–3 valves each
* common femoral, 1 valve
* external iliac, has valves only about 25% of the time
* common iliac, none
* internal iliac, none
* inferior vena cava, none
* jugular vein, 1 valve

▶ . Rumwell C, McPharlin M: *Vascular Technology: An Illustrated Review,* 2nd edition. Pasadena, Davies Publishing, 2000, p 176.

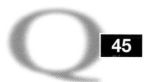

45

The bicuspid valves of the venous system are formed by folds of which of the following?

a. intima

b. media

c. adventitia

d. smooth muscle fibers

I–IV. Vascular Anatomy, Physiology, and Hemodynamics / Venous / Microscopic Anatomy (1–5%)

A **45**

A. Intima.

The venous valves are formed by folds of the venous intimal epithelium.

▶ Uflacker R: *Atlas of Vascular Anatomy—An Angiographic Approach.* Baltimore, Williams and Wilkins, 1997.

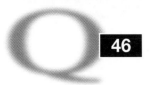

Q 46

The smallest vessels in the body are termed:

a. arterioles

b. venules

c. capillaries

d. intimas

46

C. Capillaries.

As arteries divide and become smaller and smaller they shed their outermost coat (adventitia) and become two-layered vessels known as *arterioles.* As they extend further toward the periphery, they become submillimeter in diameter and shed the tunica media. They are then single-walled vessels known as *capillaries.*

▶ Belanger AC: *Vascular Anatomy and Physiology.* Pasadena, Davies Publishing, 1999, pp 25–29.

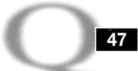 **47**

Helical flow with flow separation in the posterolateral aspect of the carotid bulb is a sign of:

a. normal flow dynamics
b. thrombosis
c. dissection
d. stenosis

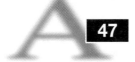

A. Normal flow dynamics.

Flow separation at the posterior wall of the carotid bulb occurs because the linear momentum of the flow is disrupted by the large sinus and sharp curve at the carotid bulb. Flow separation depends on a relatively disease-free bulb.

▶ Ku DN, Lumsden A: Blood flow patterns in cerebrovascular disease. In Bernstein EF (ed): *Noninvasive Diagnostic Techniques in Vascular Disease.* St. Louis, Mosby, 1985, pp 73–83.

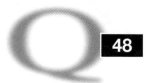

The Reynolds number describes:

a. the flow acceleration through a stenosis
b. the point at which flow becomes turbulent
c. the dampened flow proximal to a stenosis
d. the pressure drop across a hemodynamically significant stenosis

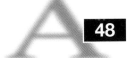

48

B. The point at which flow becomes turbulent.

The equation for the Reynolds number is $RE = Vq2r \div \eta$, where RE = Reynolds number, V = velocity, q = fluid density, r = vessel radius, and η = fluid viscosity. Turbulence begins to occur when RE exceeds 2000. Since fluid density and viscosity are constant for a given patient, the factors most responsible for creating turbulence are velocity and vessel radius.

▶ Rumwell C, McPharlin M: *Vascular Technology: An Illustrated Review,* 2nd edition. Pasadena, Davies Publishing, 2000, pp 21–22.

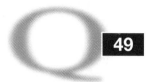

49

This spectrum was obtained with a small sample volume from the center of the internal carotid artery. Which term can be used to describe the flow depicted by this waveform?

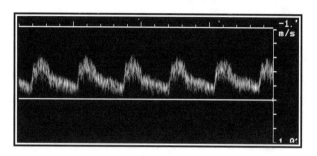

a. poststenotic turbulence

b. laminar

c. stenotic jet

d. tardus parvus

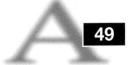

49

B. Laminar.

Laminar flow is characterized as normal, nonturbulent flow in which the blood tends to course in layers of decreasing speed from the center streamline toward the vessel wall. Laminar flow in small vessels assumes a parabolic flow profile. In larger vessels such as the common carotid artery, laminar flow assumes a more blunted or "plug" flow profile.

▶ Rumwell C, McPharlin M: *Vascular Technology: An Illustrated Review,* 2nd edition. Pasadena, Davies Publishing, 2000, pp 17, 19, 121–167.
▶ Belanger AC: *Vascular Anatomy and Physiology.* Pasadena, Davies Publishing, 1999, pp 117–125.

Which abdominal vein normally exhibits a triphasic waveform?

a. splenic vein

b. superior mesenteric vein

c. hepatic vein

d. renal vein

A **50**

C. Hepatic vein.

Q 51

Which of the following describes normal flow in the portal vein?

a. hepatopetal
b. hepatofugal
c. triphasic
d. bidirectional

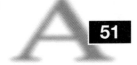

A. Hepatopetal.

Blood in the portal vein normally flows toward and into the liver. This flow direction is termed *hepatopetal*. The term *hepatofugal* describes flow coursing away from the liver in the portal vein and is a sign of advanced portal hypertension.

Q 52

Which term or terms can be used to describe the normal waveform of the hepatic veins?

a. continuous

b. unidirectional

c. triphasic

d. a and b

A 52

C. Triphasic.

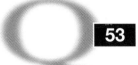

53

Which of the following veins is **NOT** a paired vein?

a. radial

b. peroneal

c. posterior tibial

d. cephalic

A 53

D. Cephalic.

Q 54

Which of the following describes the basilic vein?

a. a very small vein which joins the subclavian vein
b. a large single vein located near the brachial veins
c. a small vein located deep within the calf muscle
d. a large vein coursing lateral to the cephalic vein

DAVIES
Registry Reviews & Study Aids

54

B. A large single vein located near the brachial veins.

Q **55**

The renal arteries arise from the abdominal aorta approximately 1 cm below the:

a. inferior mesenteric artery
b. left gastric artery
c. celiac trunk
d. superior mesenteric artery

A **55**

D. Superior mesenteric artery.

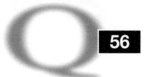

56

What is the most prevalent type of stroke?

a. ischemic

b. hemorrhagic

c. septic embolic

d. venous thrombotic

1. Cerebrovascular / Mechanisms of Disease (1–5%)

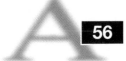

56

A. Ischemic.

Approximately 85% of strokes are ischemic in nature, with only 15% of strokes being due to intracerebral hemorrhage. Strokes caused by hemorrhage, however, account for most of the stroke fatalities.

▶ Rumwell C, McPharlin M: *Vascular Technology: An Illustrated Review,* 2nd edition. Pasadena, Davies Publishing, 2000, pp 130–136.

Q 57

Which of the following is **NOT** considered to be a risk factor for the development of stroke?

a. cigarette smoking
b. diabetes mellitus
c. cardiac arrhythmia
d. female gender

A **57**

D. Female gender.

Predisposing factors for stroke include male sex, age over 55, cigarette smoking, alcohol abuse, hypertension, diabetes mellitus, hyperlipidemia, coronary artery disease, and cardiac arrhythmia.

▶ Rumwell C, McPharlin M: *Vascular Technology: An Illustrated Review,* 2nd edition. Pasadena, Davies Publishing, 2000, pp 130–136.

Q 58

A carotid body tumor would be located:

a. between the internal and external carotid artery

b. within the internal jugular vein

c. medial to the origin of the external carotid artery

d. in the submandibular gland

58

A. Between the internal and external carotid artery.

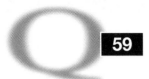

59

A fragment of atherosclerotic debris that courses distal through the vasculature until it lodges in a small vessel is a(n):

a. thrombus

b. dissection

c. embolus

d. hematoma

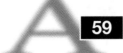

59

C. Embolus.

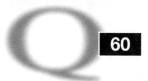

60

The arterial supply to carotid body tumors is primarily from:

a. the thyrocervical trunk

b. vasovasorum of the internal carotid artery

c. branches of the external carotid artery

d. the vertebral artery

A **60**

C. Branches of the external carotid artery.

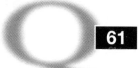

61

Innominate artery occlusion may result in reversed flow in which of the following vessels?

a. right vertebral

b. right common carotid artery

c. left vertebral artery

d. both a and b

A 61

D. Both A and B.

In the case of innominate artery occlusion, flow in the ipsilateral (right) vertebral artery will reverse to provide blood flow to the arm. If the vertebral artery can carry a sufficient volume of blood flow, carotid recovery will occur. With carotid recovery, some of the reversed flow in the vertebral will course to the common carotid artery, providing it with antegrade flow. If this is the case, the waveform profile in the common carotid will be dampened with a delay in the systolic rise time. If carotid recovery does not occur, the flow in the common carotid artery will be either bidirectional or completely retrograde, providing additional flow to the right subclavian artery. In this case the common carotid usually receives its blood supply from the ipsilateral external carotid artery.

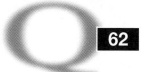

62

The biggest contributing risk factor for stroke is:

a. hypertension
b. hypercholesterolemia
c. sedentary life style
d. alcohol abuse

I. Cerebrovascular / Mechanisms of Disease (1–5%)

A 62

A. Hypertension.

Effective control of hypertension can decrease the risk of stroke by about 42%. The higher the blood pressure, the greater the risk for stroke.

▶ Kelley RE: Stroke prevention and intervention. Postgraduate Medicine 103:43–62, 1998.

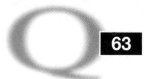

63

Which statement below is **NOT** true regarding subclavian steal?

a. most commonly occurs on the left side

b. most patients are asymptomatic

c. results from severe stenosis or occlusion of the proximal vertebral artery

d. lower blood pressure is seen in the affected arm

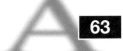

63

C. This statement—"results from severe stenosis or occlusion of the proximal vertebral artery"—is NOT true.

All other statements are correct. In subclavian steal, a severe stenosis or occlusion is present in the proximal subclavian artery. This results in retrograde flow in the ipsilateral vertebral artery. The flow is "stolen" from the contralateral vertebral artery by way of the basilar artery. Although subclavian steals occur most frequently on the left side, they are seen on the right occasionally with obstruction of the proximal right subclavian or innominate artery. Most subclavian steals are asymptomatic. When symptoms do occur, the term *subclavian steal syndrome* is used to describe the condition. The symptoms associated with subclavian steal include dizziness, vertigo, diplopia, ataxia, and bilateral blurred vision. Arm claudication or numbness is not common, but may occur in approximately one-third of patients.

▶ Ku DN, Lumsden A: Blood flow patterns in cerebrovascular disease. In Bernstein EF (ed): *Noninvasive Diagnostic Techniques in Vascular Disease.* St. Louis, Mosby, 1985, pp 73–83.

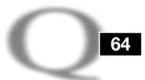 **64**

Which of the following is a complication of plaque ulceration?

a. thrombosis
b. intraplaque hemorrhage
c. embolization
d. all of the above

I. Cerebrovascular / Mechanisms of Disease (1–5%)

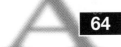

D. All of the above.

Ulceration of an atherosclerotic plaque can be described as erosion of the intimal layer over the plaque surface. This may progress to deep ulceration with embolization of plaque fragments. Thrombus formation is initiated by erosion of the plaque surface. Platelet aggregation occurs forming a thrombus directly over the ulceration. Distal embolization of thrombus fragments may be the source of TIAs. Intraplaque hemorrhage can occur as leakage of blood into the atherosclerotic plaque through the ulceration, or by rupture of the vaso vasorum.

▶ Rumwell C, McPharlin M: *Vascular Technology: An Illustrated Review,* 2nd edition. Pasadena, Davies Publishing, 2000, pp 126–135.

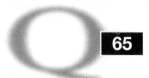

65

A 35-year-old female with a history of cystic medial necrosis presents with Horner's syndrome and left periorbital headache. Duplex carotid ultrasound reveals two channels of flow within the left common carotid artery separated by a thin echogenic flap. The most likely diagnosis is:

a. severe stenosis with plaque ulceration

b. common carotid artery dissection

c. fibromuscular dysplasia

d. Takayasu's arteritis

A **65**

B. Common carotid artery dissection.

Spontaneous dissection of the cervical carotid arteries most commonly occurs in young patients. Etiologic factors include fibromuscular dysplasia, trauma, cystic median necrosis, and Marfan's syndrome. Initially two channels of flow are present, the true lumen and a false lumen in which the blood flow tunnels between the layers of the vessel wall. This tunneling can create an intimal flap that may be visible sonographically. Dissection can result in thrombosis of the false channel, creating a long, smooth, tapering stenosis. Complete arterial thrombosis may also occur. The clinical presentation usually affects the ipsilateral eye or hemisphere. Headache is present in about 75% of patients. A headache behind the eye is particularly suggestive of ipsilateral carotid dissection.

▶ Provenzale JM: Dissection of the internal carotid and vertebral arteries: imaging features. AJR 165:1099–1104, 1995.

Q **66**

The most common location for atherosclerosis to occur in the cerebrovascular system is the:

a. the carotid bulb
b. intracranial internal carotid artery
c. left subclavian artery
d. innominate artery

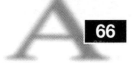

A. The carotid bulb.

▶ Rumwell C, McPharlin M: *Vascular Technology: An Illustrated Review,* 2nd edition. Pasadena, Davies Publishing, 2000, pp 121–167.

Q 67

A 65-year-old male with hypertension and diabetes presents to the vascular lab for cerebrovascular testing due to a right asymptomatic bruit. All of the following could be considered a potential source of the bruit **EXCEPT:**

a. external carotid artery stenosis

b. subclavian artery stenosis

c. common carotid artery occlusion

d. common carotid artery dissection

A 67

C. Common carotid artery occlusion.

A bruit is a result of vibration in the tissue surrounding a stenosis. A totally occluded vessel will not produce a bruit.

Q 68

A patient is referred for duplex examination to evaluate a prominent pulsatility felt in the base of the right neck. What is the most likely etiology of this physical finding?

a. CCA aneurysm
b. CCA dissection
c. excessive CCA tortuosity
d. CCA occlusion

A 68

C. Excessive CCA tortuosity.

The most common etiology of a pulsatile mass in the base of the neck is, by far, excessive tortuosity of the proximal CCA. Although an aneurysm would produce the same physical findings, aneurysms of the carotid artery is quite rare.

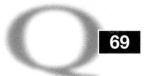

69

A unilateral temporary vision loss associated with cerebrovascular disease is known as:

a. dysphasia

b. amaurosis fugax

c. diplopia

d. ataxia

I. Cerebrovascular / Signs and Symptoms (1–5%)

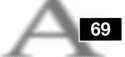

B. Amaurosis fugax.

Amaurosis fugax is frequently described by patients as "a shade coming down over one eye." It may be due to embolic process from the ipsilateral internal carotid artery. The embolus courses from the internal carotid artery to the ophthalmic artery. Other sources of emboli include the common carotid artery or heart.

▶ Rumwell C, McPharlin M: *Vascular Technology: An Illustrated Review,* 2nd edition. Pasadena, Davies Publishing, 2000, pp 133–134.

Q 70

A symptom of vertebrobasilar insufficiency is:

a. unilateral paresis

b. aphasia

c. amaurosis fugax

d. diplopia

A **70**

D. Diplopia.

Diplopia is a term for double vision and is a symptom of vertebrobasilar insufficiency.

▶ Rumwell C, McPharlin M: *Vascular Technology: An Illustrated Review,* 2nd edition. Pasadena, Davies Publishing, 2000, p 134.

Q 71

A patient presents with right arm numbness and transient loss of vision in the left eye. What vessel below is the most likely source of these symptoms?

a. right external carotid artery

b. right internal carotid artery

c. left subclavian artery

d. left internal carotid artery

I. Cerebrovascular / Signs and Symptoms (1–5%)

A **71**

D. Left internal carotid artery.

Unilateral symptoms involving the eye are associated with disease of the ipsilateral internal carotid artery, whereas unilateral symptoms involving the body are associated with the contralateral internal carotid artery.

Q 72

A 56-year-old male presents with transient numbness in the fingers of the left hand. Bilateral brachial systolic blood pressures are 130 mmHg on the right and 105 mmHg on the left. What diagnosis is suspected?

a. right subclavian artery occlusion

b. innominate artery occlusion

c. left subclavian stenosis

d. left vertebral stenosis

A 72

C. Left subclavian stenosis.

A difference of 15–20 mmHg between the brachial blood pressures suggests subclavian stenosis on the side of the lower pressure.

▶ Rumwell C, McPharlin M: *Vascular Technology: An Illustrated Review,* 2nd edition. Pasadena, Davies Publishing, 2000, p 162.

Q **73**

Neurologic symptoms that are of short duration, completely resolving in less than 24 hours, are termed:

a. CVA

b. RIND

c. TIA

d. HTN

A **73**

C. TIA.

A RIND (reversible ischemic neurologic deficit) lasts longer than a TIA (transient ischemic attack), but does completely resolve. A CVA (cerebrovascular accident) is another term for completed stroke. A stroke results in permanent damage.

▶ Rumwell C, McPharlin M: *Vascular Technology: An Illustrated Review,* 2nd edition. Pasadena, Davies Publishing, 2000, p 130.

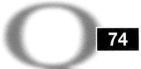

Q 74

A right-handed patient presents with expressive aphasia and left paresis. Obstruction of which of the following vessels is most likely responsible for these symptoms?

a. left internal carotid artery

b. left vertebral artery

c. basilar artery

d. right internal carotid artery

I. Cerebrovascular / Signs and Symptoms (1–5%)

A **74**

D. Right internal carotid artery.

In a right-handed person, the left hemisphere is dominant for speech. A lesion in the left middle cerebral artery may cause dysphasia or aphasia. In a left-handed person, the right hemisphere would be dominant, and a lesion in the right middle cerebral artery would produce the symptoms. The left hemisphere of the brain controls the right side of the body and vice versa. Paresis (weakness or paralysis) on one side of the body would result from an atherosclerotic lesion in the opposite side.

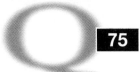

75

A 57-year-old female presents with right leg and left arm numbness. These symptoms are most closely associated with:

a. left internal carotid obstruction

b. right internal carotid obstruction

c. right common carotid obstruction

d. vertebrobasilar obstruction

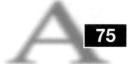

75

D. Vertebrobasilar obstruction.

Bilateral symptoms of weakness or numbness are most commonly associated with vertebrobasilar disease. This is in contrast to symptoms of cerebrovascular insufficiency, which are unilateral. Other vertebrobasilar symptoms include diplopia, bilateral visual blurring, hoarseness, dysarthria, dysphasia, ataxia, and disturbance of equilibrium. Dizziness, vertigo, and drop attacks are not considered symptoms of focal vertebrobasilar disease unless they are associated with other symptoms noted above.

▶ Rumwell C, McPharlin M: *Vascular Technology: An Illustrated Review,* 2nd edition. Pasadena, Davies Publishing, 2000, pp 130–134.

Q 76

An abnormal sound heard on auscultation caused by flow turbulence is a:

a. Bernoulli

b. bruit

c. Poiseuille

d. thrill

A 76

B. Bruit.

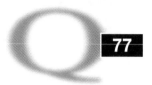

77

Auscultation of the carotid artery is best performed with:

a. the patient suspending respiration
b. the patient breathing regularly and deeply
c. the patient performing a valsalva maneuver
d. the patient in quiet respiration

A **77**

A. The patient suspending respiration.

▶ Fahey VA, White SA: Physical assessment of the vascular system. In Fahey VA (ed): *Vascular Nursing.* Philadelphia, Saunders, 1988, pp 51–68.

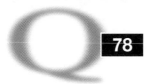

78

Hollenhorst plaques are:

a. cholesterol emboli seen on ophthalmoscopic exam within the retinal artery branches
b. complex plaques in which hemorrhage into necrotic areas has occurred
c. fibrous plaques containing an excessive amount of lipid material
d. ulcerated plaques with thrombus formation

A **78**

A. Cholesterol emboli seen on ophthalmoscopic exam within the retinal artery branches.

▶ Fahey VA, White SA: Physical assessment of the vascular system. In Fahey VA (ed): *Vascular Nursing*. Philadelphia, Saunders, 1988, pp 51–68.

79

Neurologic exam of a patient suspected of extracranial cerebrovascular disease should include:

a. evaluation of level of consciousness

b. basic comprehension

c. orientation to time and place

d. all of the above

158

A 79

D. All of the above.

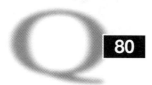

Q 80

A decreased radial pulse on one arm raises suspicion for:

a. ipsilateral subclavian artery stenosis
b. contralateral vertebral stenosis
c. ipsilateral common carotid occlusion
d. all of the above

80

A. Ipsilateral subclavian artery stenosis.

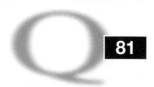

81

Why are blood pressures obtained bilaterally when evaluating a patient for cerebrovascular disease?

a. The systolic component from each arm is averaged together to determine the likelihood of cerebrovascular disease.

b. It is necessary to know both brachial pressures to rule out the presence of hypoperfusion syndrome.

c. The brachial blood pressures are compared to see if they are equal.

d. Both brachial blood pressures must be known to determine if hypertension is present.

A 81

C. The brachial blood pressures are compared to see if they are equal.

If one pressure is 15–20 mmHg less than the other, subclavian steal is suspected on the side of the lower pressure.

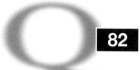
82

Which measurement is most commonly used in angiographic reports of carotid stenosis?

a. percentage area reduction
b. percentage diameter reduction

A 82

B. Percentage diameter reduction.

Percentage diameter reduction is the most common measurement parameter used in angiography as it is easily determined from a sagittal image. Percentage area reduction is calculated from a cross-sectional image.

▶ Rumwell C, McPharlin M: *Vascular Technology: An Illustrated Review,* 2nd edition. Pasadena, Davies Publishing, 2000, pp 165–166.

Q **83**

A percentage diameter reduction of 50% in a symmetric narrowing of the carotid artery most closely corresponds to what percentage area reduction?

a. 35%

b. 50%

c. 75%

d. 90%

A 83

C. 75%.

In a symmetric narrowing, a 50% diameter stenosis is approximately the same as a 75% area stenosis.

▶ Rumwell C, McPharlin M: *Vascular Technology: An Illustrated Review,* 2nd edition. Pasadena, Davies Publishing, 2000, pp 165–166.

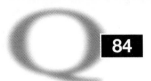

84

Percentage diameter and area reduction measurements are most accurate when obtained in which imaging plane?

a. sagittal

b. coronal

c. transverse

d. oblique

A **84**

C. Transverse.

Both percentage diameter and percentage area measurements are most accurate when obtained in the transverse scan plane. Percent stenosis measurements obtained from sagittal or coronal scan planes are easily over- or underestimated because atherosclerotic plaque is typically asymmetric. A sagittal slice obtained through the greatest dimension of asymmetric plaque will overestimate percentage stenosis, whereas a sagittal slice through the smallest dimension of the plaque will underestimate it.

▶ Rumwell C, McPharlin M: *Vascular Technology: An Illustrated Review,* 2nd edition. Pasadena, Davies Publishing, 2000, pp 165–166.
▶ Ridgway DP: *Introduction to Vascular Scanning: A Guide for the Complete Beginner,* 2nd edition. Pasadena, Davies Publishing, 1999, pp 64–65.

Q 85

The surgical removal of the atherosclerotic plaque from an artery is termed:

a. atherectomy

b. endarterectomy

c. angioplasty

d. thrombectomy

A 85

B. Endarterectomy.

Q 86

Differentiation between primary ischemic and primary hemorrhagic stroke is most readily obtained by which diagnostic test?

a. computed tomography of the brain

b. magnetic resonance angiography

c. duplex ultrasonography

d. electrocardiogram

I. Cerebrovascular / Testing (20–25%)

A 86

A. Computed tomography of the brain.

▶ Kelley RE: Stroke prevention and intervention. Postgraduate Medicine 103:43–62, 1998.

87

All of the statements below apply to continuous-wave Doppler **EXCEPT:**

a. requires both a transmitting and receiving transducer
b. shows greater spectral broadening than pulsed-wave Doppler
c. Range-gating is applied to control vessel selection.
d. The difference between the transmitted and received frequencies falls within the audible hearing range.

87

C. Range-gating is applied to control vessel selection.

Range-gating is a method applied to pulsed-wave Doppler allowing signals only from a specified depth to be processed for display. The user determines the depth of interest by placement of the sample volume. Because both the speed of sound in tissue (1540 m/sec) and the depth of interest (depth of sample volume) are known, the system can easily calculate the round trip time of the ultrasound from the transducer to the depth of interest and back again, receiving echoes only at that time.

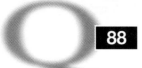

88

Loss of the spectral window with pulsed Doppler ultrasound is present with:

a. flow turbulence
b. parabolic flow
c. laminar flow
d. all of the above

A 88

A. Flow turbulence.

The spectral window is the blank area underneath systole on the spectral waveform. It is filled in or "lost" when turbulent flow creates spectral broadening. Other reasons for loss of the spectral window include overuse of Doppler gain and incorrect positioning of the sample volume outside of the center streamline (depicting signals from the vessel wall or adjacent slower-moving blood flow).

Q 89

A unilateral decrease or absence of diastolic flow in the common carotid artery is indicative of:

a. proximal disease of the aortic arch
b. poor cardiac output
c. distal obstructive disease
d. arteriovenous fistula

A 89

C. Distal obstructive disease.

A unilateral finding of decreased or absent diastolic flow in the common carotid artery is indicative of distal obstructive disease. The most likely scenario is occlusion of the cervical internal carotid artery, although high-grade stenosis of the intracranial internal carotid artery may also produce this finding.

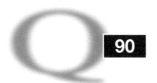

90

This image is a sagittal view of the right vertebral artery origin. Both the subclavian and the proximal vertebral artery are demonstrated. The line is pointing to what vessel?

a. ascending pharyngeal artery

b. thyrocervical trunk

c. inferior thyroid artery

d. internal mammary artery

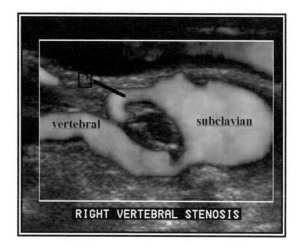

RIGHT VERTEBRAL STENOSIS

I. Cerebrovascular / Testing (20–25%)

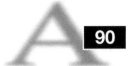

B. Thyrocervical trunk.

The thyrocervical trunk arises from the subclavian artery near the origin of the vertebral artery. The vertebral artery originates from the posterior aspect of the subclavian artery, whereas the thyrocervical trunk originates from its anterior aspect. The examiner can further differentiate the two vessels by following the vertebral artery into the transverse processes of the cervical spine. The thyrocervical trunk does not enter the spine and will course medially.

Q **91**

The frequency most commonly used for transcranial Doppler is:

a. 7.5 MHz

b. 5 MHz

c. 3 MHz

d. 2 MHz

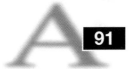

91

D. 2 MHz.

A low-frequency transducer is required for transcranial Doppler because the beam must first penetrate the temporal bone. The mean loss of power in penetrating the skull is about 80%. Higher frequencies such as those used for imaging (3–10 MHz) do not provide adequate penetration for insonating the cranial vasculature.

▶ Tegeler Ch, Eicke M: Physics and principles of transcranial Doppler ultrasonography. In Babikian VL (ed): *Transcranial Doppler Ultrasonography.* St. Louis, Mosby, 1993.

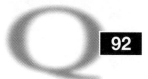

92

In conventional transcranial Doppler, the angle of insonation is assumed to be:

a. 0°

b. 45°

c. 60°

d. 90°

A **92**

A. 0°.

Because the actual vessel is not visualized with this technique, the angle of incidence is assumed to be zero degrees for calculation of velocities.

Q 93

Which testing device would be most useful in evaluation of arterial vasospasm following subarachnoid hemorrhage?

a. CW Doppler
b. OPG-Gee
c. periorbital Doppler
d. transcranial Doppler

A **93**

D. Transcranial Doppler.

One of the most widespread applications of transcranial Doppler is the evaluation of the onset, severity, and time course of arterial vasospasm caused by subarachnoid hemorrhage.

▶ Rumwell C, McPharlin M: *Vascular Technology: An Illustrated Review,* 2nd edition. Pasadena, Davies Publishing, 2000, p 157.

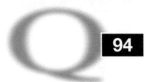

Q 94

Unilateral increased diastolic flow in the external carotid artery is commonly seen with:

a. external carotid artery stenosis

b. ipsilateral internal carotid artery occlusion

c. ipsilateral common carotid artery occlusion

d. all of the above

A 94

D. All of the above.

The external carotid artery may show increases in both systolic and diastolic flow with stenosis. This can create confusion when both the external and internal carotid arteries are stenotic. Additionally, when the external carotid artery is used as a collateral pathway through the orbit into the intracranial circulation, the diastolic flow will be increased. This can occur with extracranial occlusion of the internal and/or common carotid arteries.

Q **95**

The presence of aliasing in the spectral waveform of the internal carotid artery **ALWAYS** indicates:

a. A hemodynamically significant stenosis of the internal carotid artery.

b. An occlusion of the internal carotid artery.

c. The frequency shift exceeds ½ the system pulse repetition frequency.

d. The wall filter is set too high.

A 95

C. The frequency shift is greater than ½ the system pulse repetition frequency (PRF).

The presence or absence of aliasing in the spectral waveform cannot be used as an indicator of disease. Aliasing occurs when the received frequency shift is greater than ½ the system PRF or sampling rate. The frequency shift may be high because of small Doppler angles or high flow velocities. Aliasing may also be seen at steeper angles of incidence and lower velocities when the system PRF is set to a low value.

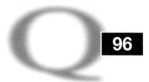

96

The point at which aliasing occurs is known as the:

a. Nyquist limit
b. Poiseuille's point
c. Bernoulli's equation
d. Reynolds number

A **96**

A. Nyquist limit.

Q 97

Which of the following is an appropriate angle for Doppler insonation of the extracranial vasculature?

a. 60°

b. 70°

c. 80°

d. 90°

A 97

A. 60°.

The Doppler angle of incidence should not exceed 60° whenever possible. As the angle of incidence exceeds 60°, the accuracy of velocity estimation diminishes. Therefore, Doppler interrogation should be performed only at angles of 60° or less.

Q 98

All of the following parameters may be used to determine the degree of stenosis in the internal carotid artery **EXCEPT**:

a. peak frequency shift

b. peak systolic velocity

c. ICA/CCA ratio

d. heart rate

A 98

D. Heart rate.

Q 99

Which letter in the illustration is pointing to end diastole?

a. A
b. B
c. C
d. D
e. E

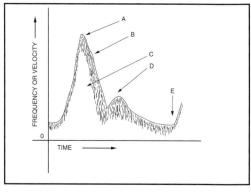

The components of the spectral display.

A 99

C. E

Q 100

Which letter represents the spectral window?

a. A
b. B
c. C
d. D
e. E

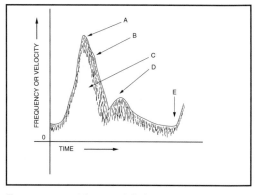

The components of the spectral display.

200

A **100**

C. C

101

Which letter is pointing to the dicrotic notch?

a. A
b. B
c. C
d. D
e. E

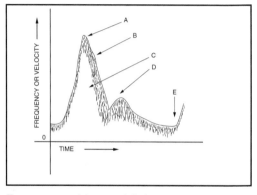

The components of the spectral display.

A **101**

D. D

Q 102

Which letter is pointing to peak systole?

a. A

b. B

c. C

d. D

e. E

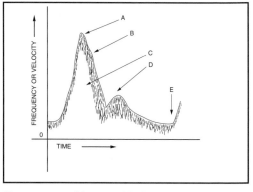

The components of the spectral display.

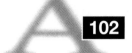

A. A

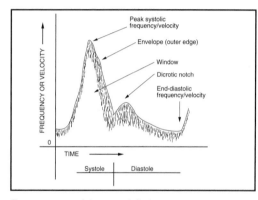

The components of the spectral display.

Q **103**

Which vessel normally exhibits a triphasic waveform?

a. common carotid artery

b. vertebral artery

c. subclavian artery

d. internal carotid artery

A **103**

C. Subclavian artery.

Q 104

On the spectral display, time is displayed on the:

a. x-axis

b. y-axis

c. z-axis

d. all of the above

104

A. x-axis.

Q 105

Which vessel normally supplies blood flow to the face and scalp?

a. external carotid artery

b. internal carotid artery

c. subclavian artery

d. thyrocervical trunk

105

A. External carotid artery.

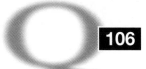

Manual tapping on the superficial temporal artery will result in the most prominent oscillations on the spectral display of the:

a. external carotid artery

b. internal carotid artery

c. subclavian artery

d. thyrocervical trunk

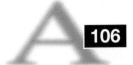

106

A. External carotid artery.

In clinical practice, the author has not found the temporal tap to be a useful technique for localizing the external carotid artery. Oscillations are frequently seen in the ICA and CCA that are as strong as or stronger than those seen in the ECA. It is better to differentiate the ICA and ECA by evaluating waveform characteristics, vessel positions, and the presence of branches. In a study published in *Radiology* in 1996, Kliewer et al. found that ". . . the temporal tap alone may not reliably distinguish the ECA from the ICA or CCA" (Radiology 201:481–484, 1996).

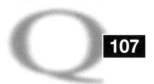

107

What term describes this waveform?

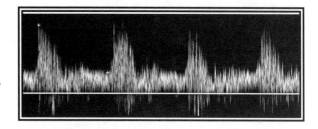

a. tardus parvus

b. spectral broadening

c. dampened

d. high resistance

DAVIES
Registry Reviews & Study Aids

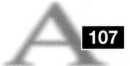

B. Spectral broadening.

On this waveform, the spectral window is "lost" or filled in. Spectral broadening represents the reflection of a wide range of frequency shifts due to interaction of the Doppler beam with a wide range of flow velocities, as in poststenotic turbulence. Spectral broadening can be thought of as a broadening of the returning spectrum of frequencies.

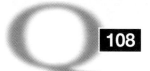

108

Using transcranial Doppler, an abnormal flow direction may be detected in the left anterior cerebral artery in cases of:

a. right internal carotid artery occlusion
b. right vertebral artery occlusion
c. left internal carotid artery occlusion
d. left external carotid artery occlusion

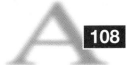
108

C. Left internal carotid artery occlusion.

Crossover collateralization may occur from one anterior cerebral artery through the anterior communicating artery to the contralateral anterior cerebral artery in cases of internal carotid artery occlusion on the same side as the reversed flow. For example, if the left internal carotid artery is occluded, the left middle cerebral artery may be supplied by reversed flow in the ipsilateral (left) anterior cerebral artery. The left anterior cerebral artery will receive its flow from the right anterior cerebral artery via the anterior communicating artery.

▶ Rumwell C, McPharlin M: *Vascular Technology: An Illustrated Review,* 2nd edition. Pasadena, Davies Publishing, 2000, pp 160–161.

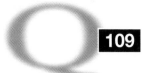

109

Waveforms obtained from an artery supplying an intracranial arteriovenous malformation will exhibit:

a. a low pulsatility index
b. absent diastolic flow
c. decreased velocities
d. triphasic flow

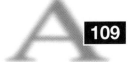
109

A. A low pulsatility index.

An artery that feeds an arteriovenous malformation will show increased velocities in both systole and diastole. The diastolic velocity especially will be increased, resulting in a waveform with very low resistance. A waveform that exhibits low resistance will have a low pulsatility index and low resistive index measurement.

▶ Rumwell C, McPharlin M: *Vascular Technology: An Illustrated Review,* 2nd edition. Pasadena, Davies Publishing, 2000, p 161.

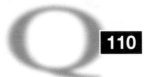

110

In transcranial Doppler, with the probe placed over the right temporal bone, flow in the right anterior cerebral artery will be:

a. oriented away from the probe
b. oriented toward the probe
c. oriented at 90° to the probe
d. The right middle cerebral artery cannot be seen from this window.

A. Oriented away from the probe.

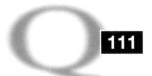

111

With transcranial Doppler, which vessel is evaluated from the foramen magnum window?

a. posterior communicating artery

b. anterior communicating artery

c. posterior cerebral artery

d. basilar artery

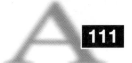

111

D. Basilar artery.

For the transforaminal (suboccipital) window, the probe is placed at the foramen magnum with the transducer angled superiorly toward the eyes. From this view, signals can be obtained from the intracranial portion of both vertebral arteries as well as the basilar artery.

▶ Tegeler Ch, Eicke M: Physics and principles of transcranial Doppler ultrasonography. In Babikian VL (ed): *Transcranial Doppler Ultrasonography.* St. Louis, Mosby, 1993.

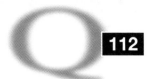

112

In transcranial Doppler, with the probe placed in the foramen magnum window, flow toward the probe in the vertebral artery is indicative of:

a.   normalcy

b.   subclavian steal

c.   basilar artery stenosis

d.   internal carotid stenosis

A 112

B. Subclavian steal.

With the probe placed at the foramen magnum window, flow in the intracranial vertebral arteries moves away from the probe. This results in a negative Doppler shift.

▶ Tegeler Ch, Eicke M: Physics and principles of transcranial Doppler ultrasonography. In Babikian VL (ed): *Transcranial Doppler Ultrasonography.* St. Louis, Mosby, 1993.

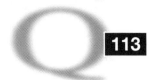

113

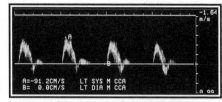

These waveforms were obtained from a 72-year-old asymptomatic male who was referred for duplex carotid ultrasound prior to undergoing surgery. The waveform at top is of the left common carotid artery. The waveform at bottom is of the right common carotid artery. Which diagnosis is most likely considering these findings?

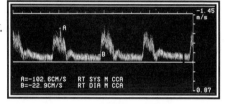

a. left arteriovenous fistula

b. right innominate occlusion

c. left internal carotid occlusion

d. right common carotid stenosis

I. Cerebrovascular / Testing (20–25%)

A 113

C. Left internal carotid occlusion.

Comparison of both common carotid artery waveforms is an important aspect of a duplex carotid study. Both sides should show a similar amount of diastolic flow. A unilateral decrease in diastole should increase suspicion for distal occlusive disease on the ipsilateral side. In other words, if the left common carotid artery shows decreased diastolic flow, distal occlusive disease involving the left internal carotid artery is suspected. Most commonly, the disease is present in the extracranial portion of the internal carotid artery near the origin, although if this portion of the internal carotid artery is normal, significant stenosis or occlusion should be suspected in the intracranial portion of the same internal carotid artery at the level of the siphon.

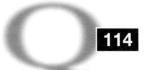

114

The presence of a mosaic pattern in the color Doppler image of the internal carotid artery most likely indicates:

a. slow flow proximal to an occlusion

b. the presence of poststenotic turbulence

c. reversed flow in the vertebral artery

d. improper color setup with the pulse repetition frequency set too high

A **114**

B. The presence of poststenotic turbulence.

A mosaic pattern on color Doppler imaging results from the reflection of a wide range of frequency shifts back to the transducer. The most likely reason for this is the wide range of velocities and flow directions present in poststenotic turbulence. Spectral broadening results in the display of a multitude of colors. Some of the colors represent aliasing caused by the higher velocities present in the poststenotic turbulence. Other colors represent reversed flow in the eddies seen distal to stenoses. The mosaic pattern alerts the examiner to the likelihood of high-grade stenosis. A similar appearance may be seen with color Doppler aliasing when the pulse repetition frequency is set too <u>low</u> for the type of flow being evaluated. In this situation the angle-corrected Doppler waveform will not reveal increased velocities or spectral broadening.

Q **115**

What technical parameters should be adjusted to increase the color Doppler sensitivity when the vessel does **NOT** fill well with color?

a. decrease color pulse repetition frequency, increase color gain, decrease color filter
b. decrease color pulse repetition frequency, increase color gain, increase color filter
c. increase color pulse repetition frequency, decrease color gain, decrease color filter
d. increase color pulse repetition frequency, decrease color gain, increase color filter

A 115

A. Decrease color pulse repetition frequency (PRF), increase color gain, decrease color filter.

When the color Doppler does not fill a vessel as expected, the system parameters should be adjusted to sensitize the color for detection of slow flow. This must be done to rule out the presence of very slow or trickle flow within a vessel. Decreasing the system PRF improves sensitivity to slow flow by increasing the time between transmitted pulses. The greater the time between pulses, the slower the flow that can be detected by the color Doppler. Increasing the color gain improves sensitivity simply by amplifying the returning echoes—similar to the volume control on a radio. Decreasing the color filter increases sensitivity because slow flow produces low-frequency shifts that are eliminated by high wall filter settings. As the color filter is decreased, lower-frequency shifts can pass through the system and be displayed on the color monitor. Unfortunately, as the color filter is lowered, low-frequency shifts from the moving vessel wall and flash artifact from patient breathing or movement are also more likely to be displayed on the color monitor and may partially obscure the vessel.

116

Power Doppler encodes which component of reflected signal?

a. frequency shift
b. velocity
c. amplitude
d. wavelength

A **116**

C. Amplitude.

Power Doppler colorizes the amplitude of the moving signals. Amplitude depends on the relative number of red blood cells passing through the beam at any given point in time. The brighter the color with power Doppler, the greater the concentration of red blood cells. The dimmer the color, the lower the concentration of red blood cells. Since the frequency shift is not displayed, power Doppler does not show flow direction or as much angle dependence as color Doppler.

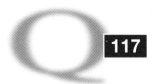

Q 117

In this B-mode picture the arrow is pointing to a dark area in the image. This dark area is caused by:

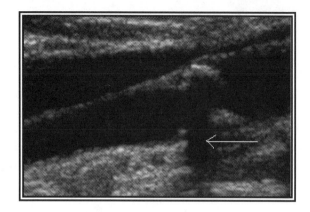

a. bad transducer element

b. inadequate amount of gel between transducer face and skin

c. ulcerated plaque

d. shadowing from calcified plaque

A 117

D. Shadowing from calcified plaque.

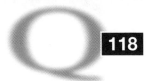

118

This waveform was most likely obtained from which vessel?

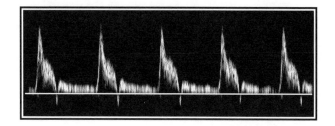

a. internal carotid artery

b. external carotid artery

c. common carotid artery

d. vertebral artery

A 118

B. External carotid artery.

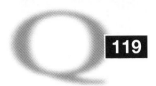

Which of the following describes
this waveform?

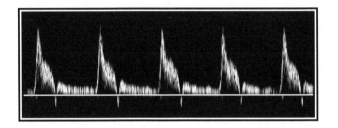

a. monophasic
b. low resistance
c. biphasic
d. high resistance

A 119

D. High resistance.

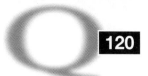

120

Which of the following is **NOT** consistent with the diagnosis of right internal carotid artery occlusion?

a. hyperemic flow in the left common carotid artery

b. low-resistance flow in the right external carotid artery

c. increased diastolic flow in the ipsilateral common carotid artery

d. debris-filled right internal carotid artery

A 120

C. Increased diastolic flow in the ipsilateral common carotid artery.

Findings that may be associated with occlusion of the internal carotid artery include:

1. Decreased or absent diastolic flow in the ipsilateral common carotid artery

2. Compensatory hyperemic flow in the contralateral common carotid artery

3. Increased diastolic flow in the ipsilateral external carotid artery when external-to-internal collateralization occurs through the orbit

4. Debris-filled internal carotid artery

5. Absence of color fill within the affected internal carotid artery when the system has been sensitized to detect slow flow

6. Absence of spectral Doppler signal within the affected internal carotid artery with the sample volume size opened to include the entire width of the vessel

7. Lack of normal pulsatility visible by B-mode in the affected internal carotid artery (a radial "jerking" motion may be detected instead)

Q 121

Duplex findings in a 58-year-old male include a systolic velocity of 58 cm/sec in the right common carotid artery and a systolic velocity of 92 cm/sec in the left common carotid artery. All of the following could be potential contributors to this finding **EXCEPT:**

a. The Doppler angle of incidence was underestimated on the right common carotid artery.

b. The Doppler angle of incidence was underestimated on the left common carotid artery.

c. There is occlusion of the right internal carotid artery.

d. There is occlusion of the innominate artery.

I. Cerebrovascular / Testing (20–25%)

A 121

B. The Doppler angle of incidence was underestimated on the left common carotid artery.

Probably the most common error in performance of a duplex ultrasound study is improper measurement of the Doppler angle of incidence. When proper measurement is performed, the angle correct cursor is aligned parallel to the vessel wall at the point of Doppler sampling. The resultant angle should be 60° or less. If the angle of incidence exceeds 60°, the velocity estimation may be inaccurate. Similarly, if the angle correct cursor is incorrectly aligned, the velocity estimation will be inaccurate. Overestimation of the angle of incidence will result in overestimation of the velocity and underestimation of the angle of incidence will result in underestimation of the velocity.

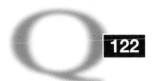

122

What is the most likely explanation for this waveform, which was obtained in the proximal left internal carotid artery of a 62-year-old male?

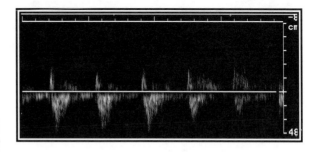

a. reversed internal carotid artery flow due to ipsilateral external carotid artery occlusion

b. reversed flow in a stump proximal to internal carotid artery occlusion

c. improper setup of the system pulse repetition frequency

d. reversed flow in the internal carotid artery due to ipsilateral vertebral artery occlusion

A 122

B. Reversed flow in a stump proximal to internal carotid artery occlusion.

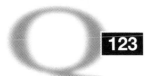

123

The top waveform was obtained from the mid left internal carotid artery and the bottom waveform from the mid right internal carotid artery. What is the most likely diagnosis?

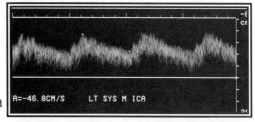

A=-46.8CM/S   LT SYS M ICA

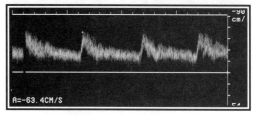

A=-63.4CM/S

a. distal stenosis in the left internal carotid artery

b. innominate occlusion

c. high-grade stenosis of the proximal left common carotid artery

d. distal stenosis in the right internal carotid artery

DAVIES
Registry Reviews & Study Aids

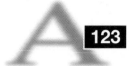

A **123**

C. High-grade stenosis of the proximal left common carotid artery.

   With significant proximal stenosis, the waveforms obtained distal to the disease may show dampening of the systolic component with a delayed systolic rise time. With significant disease distal to the site of sampling, the diastolic component will be dampened because of the increased resistance to flow toward the obstruction.

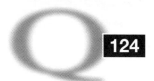

124

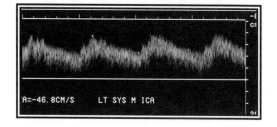

What term can be used to describe this waveform?

a. high resistance

b. spectral broadening

c. tardus parvus

d. triphasic

A 124

C. Tardus parvus. See answer to question 268.

Q 125

Overestimation of the degree of stenosis in the internal carotid artery may be due to all of the following **EXCEPT:**

a. increased velocities contralateral to an occlusion

b. overestimation of the angle of incidence

c. improper location of the sample volume proximal to the stenosis

d. vessel tortuosity

A 125

C. Improper location of the sample volume proximal to the stenosis.

Doppler samples obtained proximal to the point of stenosis will produce lower velocities than those obtained at the narrowing, resulting in underestimation of the degree of stenosis. Overestimation of the Doppler angle will result in overestimation of the velocity. Vessel tortuosities may result in overestimation or underestimation of stenosis because accurate measurement of the Doppler angle is difficult. Velocities contralateral to occlusion may be increased due to compensatory flow. Thus, stenosis is likely to be overestimated when it occurs contralateral to an occlusion.

▶ Rumwell C, McPharlin M: *Vascular Technology: An Illustrated Review,* 2nd edition. Pasadena, Davies Publishing, 2000, pp 150–157.

126

An angiogram shows an embolus lodged in the right middle cerebral artery. The source of the embolus could be from:

a. ulcerated plaque in the right internal carotid artery

b. complex plaque in the right external carotid artery

c. nonvalvular atrial fibrillation

d. a and c only

DAVIES
Registry Reviews & Study Aids

126

D. A and C only.

The external carotid artery does not feed into the middle cerebral artery, and so complex plaque at this site cannot be a source of emboli for that artery. Ulcerated plaque in the ipsilateral internal or common carotid artery may produce emboli that travel into the middle cerebral artery. Cardiac disease also poses a risk for embolic stroke: Nonvalvular atrial fibrillation and vegetations on valves, among other things, can produce emboli.

▶ Rumwell C, McPharlin M: *Vascular Technology: An Illustrated Review,* 2nd edition. Pasadena, Davies Publishing, 2000, pp 121–122.

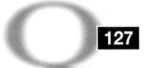

127

The most commonly used artery for catheter insertion to perform arteriography of the carotid circulation is the:

a. superficial femoral artery

b. common femoral artery

c. axillary artery

d. brachial artery

A **127**

B. Common femoral artery.

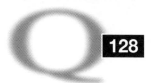

Which of the following cannot be determined from an arteriogram?

a. percent diameter stenosis
b. reversed flow in the vertebral
c. arterial dissection
d. flow turbulence

A **128**

D. Flow turbulence.

Arteriography shows a two-dimensional view of the anatomy from which percentage diameter stenosis can be measured. Reversed flow can be detected with delayed films, and dissection can be seen as well. Since hemodynamics cannot be evaluated with this technique, flow turbulence is not detected.

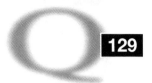

129

Blood from the deep venous system will back up into the superficial system when:

a. perforating veins are competent
b. perforating veins are incompetent
c. normal venous hemodynamics are present
d. the calf muscles contract

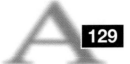 **129**

B. Perforating veins are incompetent.

With incompetent perforating veins, blood will flow retrograde from the deep venous system into the superficial venous system, increasing venous pressure.

▶ Rumwell C, McPharlin M: *Vascular Technology: An Illustrated Review,* 2nd edition. Pasadena, Davies Publishing, 2000, p 184.

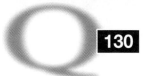

130

Elevated peripheral venous pressure results in:

a. edema

b. decreased arterial resistance

c. lymphangitis

d. dependent rubor

A 130

A. Edema.

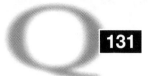

131

The greatest clinical danger from venous thrombosis is:

a. pulmonary embolism

b. superficial venous obstruction

c. venous hypertension

d. incompetent valves

A 131

A. Pulmonary embolism.

132

Virchow's triad consists of three factors that are significant in the development of venous thrombosis. These are:

a. stasis, hypercoagulability, extrinsic compression
b. hypercoagulability, cancer, stasis
c. stasis, extrinsic compression, trauma
d. trauma, stasis, hypercoagulability

A 132

D. Trauma, stasis, hypercoagulability.

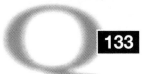

133

In the lower extremity, the most common place for thrombus to begin is the:

a. soleal sinuses

b. perforating veins

c. Boyd's veins

d. Dodd's veins

A 133

A. Soleal sinuses.

In the lower extremity, the soleal sinuses of the calf muscle are the most common site of thrombus formation. See also answer to question 266.

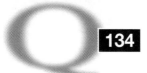

134

Which of the following is **NOT** a predisposing factor for the development of venous thrombosis?

a. pregnancy

b. bone fracture

c. a long airplane trip

d. daily use of aspirin

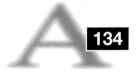

D. Daily use of aspirin.

Pregnancy, bone fracture, or a long airplane trip all can lead to stasis, which is one of the factors in Virchow's triad leading to venous thrombosis.

Q 135

Which statement is **TRUE** regarding incompetent venous valves?

a. Incompetent valves promote flow toward the heart.

b. Incompetent valves result in decreased venous pressure.

c. Incompetent valves may lead to hemosiderin deposition.

d. Incompetent valves decrease the likelihood of venous thrombosis.

A 135

C. Incompetent valves may lead to hemosiderin deposition.

Incompetent venous valves may result in increased venous pressure as blood flows retrograde (away from the heart). This produces stasis and the increased likelihood of the development of venous thrombosis. Red blood cells and fibrinogen may leak into the surrounding tissue, leading to hemosiderin deposition. This causes the brawny skin changes that are associated with chronic venous disease.

▶ Oliver MA: Clinical evaluation. In Talbot SR, Oliver MA: *Techniques of Venous Imaging.* Pasadena, Davies Publishing, 1992, pp 27–36.

Q 136

The most common cause of upper extremity venous thrombus is:

a. weight lifting

b. blunt trauma

c. pregnancy

d. intravenous catheters and lines

A **136**

D. Intravenous catheters and lines.

Upper extremity venous thrombosis, once rare, has become much more common due to increased use of intravenous lines and catheters during hospital stays.

Q 137

Primary varicose veins form as a result of:

a. incompetent or absent venous valves

b. Baker's cysts

c. lymphedema

d. venous ulcers

A 137

A. Incompetent or absent venous valves.

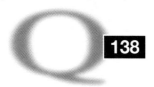

138

Lymphedema is a result of:

a. deep venous thrombosis
b. incompetent venous valves
c. impaired transport of lymph
d. chronic venous insufficiency

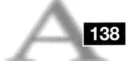

138

C. Impaired transport of lymph.

There is much that is not understood about the etiology of lymphedema. Although clinically it is easily confused with venous thrombosis because of the associated limb swelling, lymphedema is the result of the impaired transport of lymph. This impairment may be caused by a malfunction of lymph nodes, too few lymph nodes, obstructed lymph node pathway, or fluid overload.

▶ Dixon MB, Bergan JJ: Lymphedema. In Fahey VA (ed): *Vascular Nursing*. Philadelphia, W. B. Saunders Co, 1988, pp 33–47.

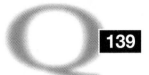

Q 139

Which statement is **NOT** true regarding varicose veins?

a. Primary varicose veins occur in the greater and lesser saphenous system.

b. Secondary varicose veins result from obstruction of the deep venous system.

c. Secondary varicose veins are the most common type of varicose veins.

d. Stasis in dilated, tortuous varicose veins can lead to thrombosis.

A 139

C. This statement—"secondary varicose veins are the most common type of varicose veins"—is NOT true.

Primary varicose veins are the most common type of varicose veins.

▶ Fahey VA: Chronic venous disease. In Fahey VA (ed): *Vascular Nursing*. Philadelphia, Saunders, 1988, pp 369–391.

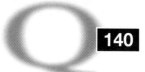

140

Phelgmasia cerulea dolens is a serious condition associated with:

a. cyanosis

b. iliofemoral deep venous thrombosis

c. decreased arterial inflow due to severely reduced venous outflow

d. all of the above

A 140

D. All of the above.

▶ Rumwell C, McPharlin M: *Vascular Technology: An Illustrated Review,* 2nd edition. Pasadena, Davies Publishing, 2000, p 185.

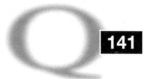

141

Blue toe syndrome is caused by:

a. venous thrombosis of the pedal veins

b. hyperemic flow from arteriovenous fistulas

c. congenital absence of the dorsalis pedis artery

d. embolization from proximal arteries

A **141**

D. Embolization from proximal arteries.

▶ Rumwell C, McPharlin M: *Vascular Technology: An Illustrated Review,* 2nd edition. Pasadena, Davies Publishing, 2000, p 113.

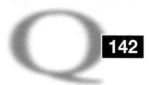

142

The most common features of symptomatic venous thrombosis are:

a. pain and tenderness
b. ulceration
c. discoloration
d. Homan's sign

A **142**

A. Pain and tenderness.

▶ Oliver MA: Clinical evaluation. In Talbot SR, Oliver MA: *Techniques of Venous Imaging.* Pasadena, Davies Publishing, 1992, pp 27–36.

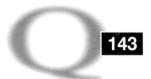

Q 143

Symptoms of pulmonary embolism include all of the following **EXCEPT:**

a. dyspnea

b. chest pain

c. tachycardia

d. claudication

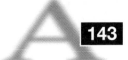

143

D. Claudication.

A venous thrombus that has embolized to the lungs is known as a pulmonary embolus. Pulmonary embolism may be symptomatic or asymptomatic and is potentially fatal. Symptoms of pulmonary embolism include chest pain, dyspnea, tachycardia, and tachypnea.

▶ Oliver MA: Clinical evaluation. In Talbot SR, Oliver MA: *Techniques of Venous Imaging.* Pasadena, Davies Publishing, 1992, pp 27–36.

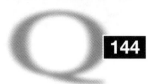

Homan's sign is:

a. a highly specific sign for lower extremity venous thrombosis
b. a highly specific sign for upper extremity venous thrombosis
c. calf discomfort on passive dorsiflexion
d. numbness of the digits with hyperextension of an extremity

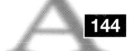

144

C. Calf discomfort on passive dorsiflexion.

Homan's sign is a nonspecific and insensitive sign for venous thrombosis and should not be used.

▶ Oliver MA: Clinical evaluation. In Talbot SR, Oliver MA: *Techniques of Venous Imaging.* Pasadena, Davies Publishing, 1992, pp 27–36.

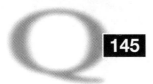

145

A sign of chronic venous insufficiency is:

a. dyspnea
b. shooting pains in the extremity
c. numbness
d. hyperpigmentation

A **145**

D. Hyperpigmentation.

The hyperpigmentation occurs as a result of the breakdown of red blood cells into hemosiderin deposits. (See also answer to question 135.) Shooting pains is a more common symptom of neuro-muscular problems. Dyspnea is a symptom of pulmonary embolism, which is more common in acute cases of venous thrombosis. Numbness is more commonly associated with arterial insufficiency.

146

Iliac vein thrombosis most likely results in:

a.   unilateral swelling isolated to the calf

b.   bilateral calf vein swelling

c.   unilateral swelling of the entire lower extremity

d.   no swelling of either extremity

A **146**

C. Unilateral swelling of the entire lower extremity.

▶ Fahey VA, White SA: Physical assessment of the vascular system. In Fahey VA (ed): *Vascular Nursing*. Philadelphia, Saunders, 1988, pp 51–68.

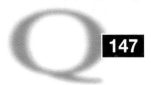

147

Inferior vena cava thrombosis most likely results in:

a. swelling of the right lower extremity only
b. bilateral swelling of the lower extremities
c. unilateral calf vein swelling
d. abdominal cavity swelling

A 147

B. Bilateral swelling of the lower extremities.

Q 148

A 42-year-old female presents with a gradual onset of asymptomatic right lower extremity swelling which began at the dorsum of the foot and gradually included the whole leg. These findings are most likely associated with:

a. acute deep venous thrombosis involving the popliteal vein

b. lymphedema

c. Baker's cyst

d. acute superficial venous thrombosis involving the greater saphenous vein

A 148

B. Lymphedema.

Lymphedema may be very difficult to differentiate from deep venous thrombosis clinically. The gradual onset of swelling over a period of several months, which begins at the dorsum of the foot and is not associated with other symptoms, is characteristic of lymphedema. Acute DVT involving the popliteal vein would produce swelling in the calf associated with pain or tenderness that was not of a gradual onset. Superficial venous thrombosis of the greater saphenous vein would most likely produce pain and tenderness over the thrombus site. A Baker's cyst will not cause swelling of the entire lower extremity.

▶ Dixon MB, Bergan JJ: Lymphedema. In Fahey VA (ed): *Vascular Nursing*. Philadelphia, W. B. Saunders Co, 1988, pp 33–47.

Q 149

Which finding is **NOT** associated with venous ulcers?

a.   brawny discoloration

b.   shiny skin

c.   location near medial malleolus

d.   irregular borders

A **149**

B. Shiny skin.

Venous ulcers tend to have a brawny discoloration. Arterial ulcers exhibit shiny skin with loss of hair.

▶ Rumwell C, McPharlin M: *Vascular Technology: An Illustrated Review,* 2nd edition. Pasadena, Davies Publishing, 2000, pp 185–186.

Q 150

Which of the following is the most important in physical examination of the venous system?

a. auscultation

b. palpation

c. inspection

d. a and b

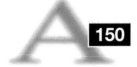

C. Inspection.

Because venous sounds are not audible with a stethoscope, auscultation is not helpful except in cases of arteriovenous fistula. Palpation only offers minimal information in evaluation of the venous system. Inspection of the extremities, however, is very important. The patient suspected of venous disease is inspected for limb swelling, ulceration, color changes, and cellulitis.

Q 151

Persistent inflammation of the skin around the ankle with a tendency toward a brown pigmentation is known as:

a. cyanosis

b. pallor

c. stasis dermatitis

d. phlegmasia

A 151

C. Stasis dermatitis.

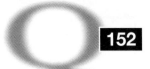

152

Which physical finding is more frequently seen with arterial insufficiency rather than venous stasis?

a. red or blue skin

b. pallor

c. brown skin discoloration

d. induration

A **152**

B. Pallor.

All of these findings may be seen with venous stasis. Pallor is more common in arterial insufficiency but may be seen with venous stasis due to arterial spasm in acute iliofemoral deep venous thrombosis.

▶ Oliver MA: Clinical evaluation. In Talbot SR, Oliver MA: *Techniques of Venous Imaging.* Pasadena, Davies Publishing, 1992, pp 27–36.

153

A condition characterized by severe swelling of the leg without redness or cyanosis secondary to acute iliofemoral deep venous thrombosis is:

a. phlegmasia alba dolens

b. pitting edema

c. lipedema

d. cellulitis

A 153

A. Phlegmasia alba dolens.

This serious condition is caused by arterial spasms secondary to the extensive, acute deep iliofemoral venous thrombosis.

▶ Rumwell C, McPharlin M: *Vascular Technology: An Illustrated Review,* 2nd edition. Pasadena, Davies Publishing, 2000, p 185.

Q **154**

Varicose veins are best visualized with the patient in which position?

a. standing

b. supine

c. Trendelenburg

d. prone

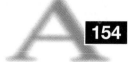

154

A. Standing.

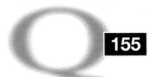

155

Which is **NOT** a limitation of CW Doppler evaluation for deep venous thrombosis?

a. Partial thrombus may not be detected.
b. Well-collateralized thrombosis may show normal flow patterns.
c. Venous incompetence cannot be detected.
d. Inaccurate results may be obtained with a bifed venous system.

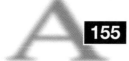

C. This statement—"venous incompetence cannot be detected"—is NOT true. CW Doppler can be used to evaluate for venous incompetence.

▶ Rumwell C, McPharlin M: *Vascular Technology: An Illustrated Review,* 2nd edition. Pasadena, Davies Publishing, 2000, p 197.

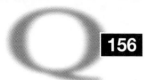

156

In the lower extremity, maximum flow return in the venous system is present with:

a. inspiration

b. expiration

c. valsalva maneuver

d. release of distal compression

A 156

B. Expiration.

In the lower extremity, flow in the venous system is diminished or absent during inspiration and maximal during expiration. Flow may be increased by release of proximal compression or distal augmentation.

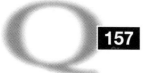

157

A pulsatile venous signal is associated with:

a. congestive heart failure

b. deep venous thrombosis

c. varicose veins

d. pulmonary embolism

A **157**

A. Congestive heart failure.

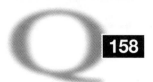

158

Detection of venous flow with compression proximal (closer to the heart) to the probe indicates:

a. venous thrombosis between the compression and site of Doppler interrogation

b. absence of venous thrombosis above the level of compression

c. valvular incompetence with reflux between the augmentation and the Doppler interrogation

d. functional valves between the augmentation and the Doppler interrogation

A 158

C. Valvular incompetence with reflux between the augmentation and the Doppler interrogation.

If augmentation of the Doppler signal occurs with proximal limb compression, then blood flow is being forced backward through the vein under examination. If there is a valve between the two points, valvular incompetence and reflux are indicated.

▶ Rumwell C, McPharlin M: *Vascular Technology: An Illustrated Review,* 2nd edition. Pasadena, Davies Publishing, 2000, pp 199–200.

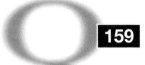

159

A continuous venous signal obtained with CW Doppler is commonly seen with:

a. normality

b. congestive heart failure

c. fluid overload

d. collateral flow

A 159

D. Collateral flow.

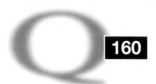

160

A normal Doppler response for the femoral vein during a Valsalva maneuver is:

a. augmentation
b. increased pulsatility of the venous signal
c. no change in flow
d. cessation of flow

DAVIES
Registry Reviews & Study Aids

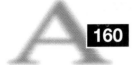

A **160**

D. Cessation of flow.

A Valsalva maneuver is performed by the patient taking in a breath and then bearing down as if to have a bowel movement. This maneuver can be performed to evaluate for valvular competency. Normally, flow ceases during a Valsalva maneuver. If flow persists or increases, the valves between the groin and the area of interrogation are incompetent.

▶ Rumwell C, McPharlin M: *Vascular Technology: An Illustrated Review,* 2nd edition. Pasadena, Davies Publishing, 2000, pp 181, 200.

Q 161

Augmentation of the Doppler signal in the femoral vein with calf compression is indicative of:

a. reflux

b. incompetent valves

c. deep venous thrombosis in the popliteal vein

d. normality

A 161

D. Normality.

Q 162

For duplex evaluation of the lower extremity veins, the patient should be positioned:

a. Trendelenburg

b. reversed Trendelenburg

c. decubitus

d. standing

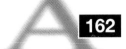

162

B. Reversed Trendelenburg.

In a reversed Trendelenburg position, the bed is tilted 10–20° with the feet lower than the head. This position promotes pooling of the blood within the veins, enlarging them and making them easier to visualize.

▶ Rumwell C, McPharlin M: *Vascular Technology: An Illustrated Review,* 2nd edition. Pasadena, Davies Publishing, 2000, p 201.

Q 163

What vessels are seen with duplex ultrasound at the level of the inguinal ligament?

a. external iliac vein, internal iliac vein

b. femoral vein, superficial femoral artery, deep femoral artery

c. external iliac vein, internal iliac artery

d. common femoral vein, common femoral artery

A 163

D. Common femoral vein, common femoral artery.

Q 164

The saphenofemoral junction is identified by duplex sonography at:

a. the level of the knee
b. the mid thigh
c. in the adductor canal
d. near the inguinal ligament

A **164**

D. Near the inguinal ligament.

Q 165

If the greater saphenous vein is **NOT** identified at the appropriate location, the examiner should:

a. use a posterior approach

b. use a lateral approach

c. decrease probe pressure

d. increase probe pressure

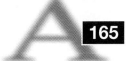

165

C. Decrease probe pressure.

Too much probe pressure is the mistake most commonly responsible for a failure to visualize the greater saphenous or other superficial veins. These vessels are easily compressed by the weight of the probe resting on the skin.

▶ Talbot SR: Venous imaging technique. In Talbot SR, Oliver MA: *Techniques of Venous Imaging.* Pasadena, Davies Publishing, 1992, pp 59–118.

166

Which veins located within the calf muscle are a common site of thrombus formation?

a. geniculate veins

b. Hunter's veins

c. soleal veins

d. anterior tibial veins

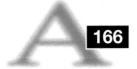

C. Soleal veins.

The soleal veins are located in the calf within the soleal muscle. They are a common site of thrombus formation. The soleal veins do not communicate with the superficial venous system; they empty into either the peroneal veins or the posterior tibial veins.

▶ Talbot SR: Venous imaging technique. In Talbot SR, Oliver MA: *Techniques of Venous Imaging.* Pasadena, Davies Publishing, 1992, pp 59–118.

Q 167

With duplex sonography, the main purpose of probe compression is to:

a. rule out incompetent valves
b. rule out the presence of thrombus
c. differentiate between superficial and deep veins
d. differentiate between veins and arteries

A 167

B. Rule out the presence of thrombus.

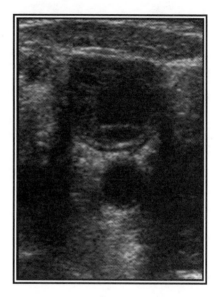

Q 168

This image shows a thrombosed vein adjacent to the common carotid artery. What vein is being imaged?

a. subclavian vein

b. external jugular vein

c. internal jugular vein

d. innominate vein

DAVIES
Registry Reviews & Study Aids

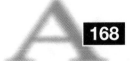

C. Internal jugular vein.

The internal jugular vein courses with the common carotid artery. The external jugular vein does not accompany an artery.

▶ Talbot SR: Venous imaging technique. In Talbot SR, Oliver MA: *Techniques of Venous Imaging.* Pasadena, Davies Publishing, 1992, pp 59–118.

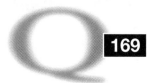

169

Which color Doppler pattern is seen with valvular incompetency?

a. Color Doppler cannot detect valvular incompetency.
b. There is no change in color with proximal compression.
c. A reversal of color is seen with distal compression.
d. A reversal of color is seen with Valsalva maneuver.

A 169

D. A reversal of color is seen with Valsalva maneuver.

Both proximal compression and the Valsalva maneuver can be used to rule out valvular incompetency. If a reversal of color is seen (from red to blue or blue to red) with either proximal compression or a Valsalva maneuver, valvular incompetency is suspected.

▶ Talbot SR: Venous imaging technique. In Talbot SR, Oliver MA: *Techniques of Venous Imaging*. Pasadena, Davies Publishing, 1992, pp 59–118.

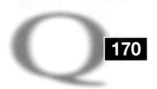

Q 170

A technologist performing a venous study on the lower extremity notes that color Doppler does **NOT** fill the calf veins spontaneously. What technical factors could be adjusted to improve color saturation?

a. increase color filter, decrease color pulse repetition frequency, increase color gain

b. decrease color filter, decrease color pulse repetition frequency, increase color gain

c. decrease color filter, increase color pulse repetition frequency, decrease color gain

d. increase color filter, increase color pulse repetition frequency, increase color gain

DAVIES
Registry Reviews & Study Aids

A 170

B. Decrease color filter, decrease color pulse repetition frequency (PRF), increase color gain.

The flow in the calf veins is very slow and may not be detected at default color settings. To sensitize the color system to detect slow moving blood flow, both the color PRF and the wall filter should be decreased. Increasing the color gain will amplify the signal that is received and increase the display of color.

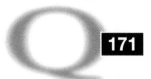

171

Probe compression in venous ultrasound is best performed in:

a. B-mode in a transverse orientation

b. B-mode in a sagittal orientation

c. color mode in a transverse orientation

d. color mode in a sagittal orientation

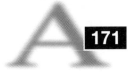

171

A. B-mode in a transverse orientation.

▶ Oliver MA: Doppler color flow imaging. In Talbot SR, Oliver MA: *Techniques of Venous Imaging.* Pasadena, Davies Publishing, 1992, pp 119–134.

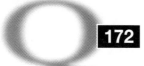

Q 172

Which characteristics below are associated with acute thrombus?

a. poorly attached, dilated vein, brightly echogenic, irregular borders
b. large collateral veins, contracted vein, brightly echogenic, irregular borders
c. poorly attached, dilated vein, hypoechoic, smooth borders
d. contracted vein, large collateral veins, hypoechoic, poorly attached

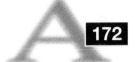

172

C. Poorly attached, dilated vein, hypoechoic, smooth borders.

These are all characteristics of acute thrombosis as opposed to chronic thrombosis. Other characteristics of acute thrombosis include a spongy texture and incompressible vein.

▶ Talbot SR: Thrombus identification and characteristics. In Talbot SR, Oliver MA: *Techniques of Venous Imaging.* Pasadena, Davies Publishing, 1992, pp 37–58.

Q 173

Which characteristics below are associated with chronic thrombus?

a. poorly attached, dilated vein, brightly echogenic, irregular borders
b. large collateral veins, contracted vein, brightly echogenic, irregular borders
c. poorly attached, dilated vein, hypoechoic, smooth borders
d. contracted vein, large collateral veins, hypoechoic, poorly attached

A **173**

B. Large collateral veins, contracted vein, brightly echogenic, irregular borders.

▶ Talbot SR: Thrombus identification and characteristics. In Talbot SR, Oliver MA: *Techniques of Venous Imaging.* Pasadena, Davies Publishing, 1992, pp 37–58.

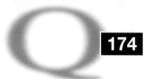

174

Coaptation of the supraclavicular subclavian vein is best performed by:

a. probe compression
b. Valsalva maneuver
c. distal limb compression
d. patient takes in quick, deep breath

A 174

D. Patient takes in quick, deep breath.

Because the subclavian vein is usually inaccessible to probe compression, coaptation can be performed by having the patient take in a quick, deep breath (sniff). If the walls are seen to completely coapt, that portion of the vein is judged to be thrombus-free.

▶ Talbot SR: Venous imaging technique. In Talbot SR, Oliver MA: *Techniques of Venous Imaging.* Pasadena, Davies Publishing, 1992, pp 59–118.

Q 175

A patient referred to the vascular lab presents with bilateral lower extremity edema and nephrotic syndrome. Thrombus is suspected within what vessel?

a. portal vein

b. left iliac vein

c. inferior vena cava

d. splenic vein

A **175**

C. Inferior vena cava.

IVC thrombus may produce bilateral leg swelling and recurrent pulmonary embolus. Nephrotic syndrome may occur if the thrombus is located at the level of the renal veins.

176

Which is an advantage of color Doppler imaging over B-mode imaging alone in evaluation of the venous system?

a. Recanalized thrombi are more readily apparent.

b. Partially occluding thrombi are better detected.

c. Venous collaterals are more readily visualized.

d. All of the above.

A 176

D. All of the above.

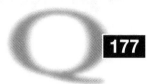

177

A normal Doppler response for the femoral vein immediately following a Valsalva maneuver is:

a. augmentation

b. increased pulsatility of the venous signal

c. no change in flow

d. cessation of flow

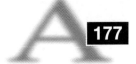

177

A. Augmentation.

Immediately following a Valsalva maneuver, the venous flow will be augmented as blood can now course proximal.

▶ Rumwell C, McPharlin M: *Vascular Technology: An Illustrated Review,* 2nd edition. Pasadena, Davies Publishing, 2000, p 200.

Q **178**

A 48-year-old male is referred to the vascular lab to rule out the presence of a Baker's cyst. What anatomy would be imaged in this study?

a. Morrison's pouch
b. Hunter's canal
c. popliteal fossa
d. subclavicular area

A **178**

C. Popliteal fossa.

A Baker's cyst is seen as an anechoic area or area of mixed echogenicity in the popliteal fossa. It is separate from the artery and vein and does not fill with color Doppler. Also known as popliteal cysts, Baker's cysts are collections of synovial fluid in a sac posterior to the knee, although they may dissect down into the calf area. They can be quite painful.

▶ Talbot SR: Thrombus identification and characteristics. In Talbot SR, Oliver MA: *Techniques of Venous Imaging.* Pasadena, Davies Publishing, 1992, pp 37–58.

Q 179

Which vessels would be the most difficult to coapt with probe compression in cross section?

a. confluence of the femoral and saphenous vein
b. posterior tibial vein above the medial malleolus
c. superficial femoral vein at the adductor canal
d. peroneal veins in the mid calf

A 179

C. Superficial femoral vein at the adductor canal.

The femoral vein is sometimes difficult to visualize and/or compress at the level of the adductor canal. Compression can be made easier by the simple technique of placing one hand behind the leg and pressing upward while also pushing down with the other hand on the probe. Color Doppler can also be useful here to confirm patency of the vein.

Q 180

On a duplex examination of a 45-year-old male, a thrombus is seen in one of the gastrocnemius veins. Propagation of this thrombus would most likely involve which vein?

a. common femoral
b. anterior tibial
c. popliteal
d. soleal

A 180

C. Popliteal.

The gastrocnemius veins are located around the knee and drain into the popliteal vein.

Q 181

During expiration, what is the effect on a Doppler waveform obtained in the axillary vein?

a. no effect

b. augmentation

c. reverses

d. stops

A 181

D. Stops.

During expiration, venous flow from the lower extremities increases, whereas venous flow in the upper extremities stops.

▶ Rumwell C, McPharlin M: *Vascular Technology: An Illustrated Review,* 2nd edition. Pasadena, Davies Publishing, 2000, p 181.

Q **182**

A venous refill time that is < 20 seconds without a tourniquet and < 20 seconds with a tourniquet applied below the knee is consistent with:

a. insufficiency of the deep and superficial systems

b. normality

c. reflux in the greater saphenous vein

d. reflux in the lesser saphenous vein

A **182**

A. Insufficiency of the deep and superficial systems.

A normal venous refill time (VRT) is ≥ 20 seconds. A VRT of < 20 seconds without the tourniquet in conjunction with a VRT > 20 seconds with a tourniquet below the knee is consistent with reflux in the lesser saphenous vein. A VRT of < 20 seconds without the tourniquet in conjunction with a VRT > 20 seconds with a tourniquet above the knee is consistent with reflux in the greater saphenous vein.

▶ Rumwell C, McPharlin M: *Vascular Technology: An Illustrated Review,* 2nd edition. Pasadena, Davies Publishing, 2000, p 196.

Q 183

This Doppler waveform was obtained in the femoral vein. The arrow is pointing to an augmented portion of the spectrum. This could be caused by:

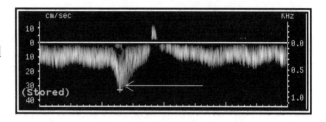

a. distal limb compression
b. release of distal limb compression
c. proximal limb compression
d. Valsalva maneuver

A

183

A. Distal limb compression.

With distal limb compression, blood is forced rapidly upstream past the point of Doppler sampling, thereby augmenting flow. This would not occur with release of the distal limb compression. Flow would cease with proximal limb compression or Valsalva maneuver.

▶ Rumwell C, McPharlin M: *Vascular Technology: An Illustrated Review,* 2nd edition. Pasadena, Davies Publishing, 2000, p 199.

Q 184

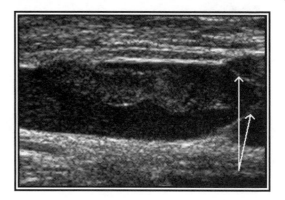

This image was obtained in the internal jugular vein of a 34-year-old female. What is the most likely diagnosis?

a. acute thrombus

b. chronic thrombus

c. rouleaux formation without thrombus

d. valvular incompetence

184

A. Acute thrombus.

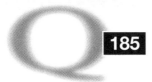

185

The arrows in this image point to:

a. rouleaux formation

b. valve leaflets

c. recanalized channels through thrombus

d. reverberation artifacts

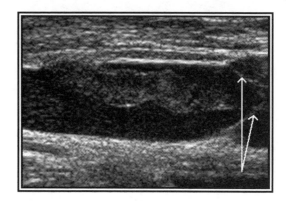

185

B. Valve leaflets.

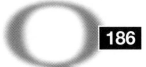

186

In contrast venography of the lower extremity, the radiopaque material is injected into veins in the:

a. foot

b. calf

c. inguinal region

d. arm

A 186

A. Foot.

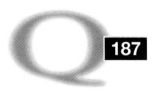

187

In contrast venography, which finding would indicate the presence of a thrombus?

a. contrast extravasation
b. filling defect
c. increase in opacity
d. none of the above

187

B. Filling defect.

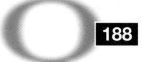

Contrast venography is **NOT** frequently performed today because:

a. It is inaccurate.

b. There is a very high rate of severe allergic reactions.

c. Duplex scanning is an accurate, noninvasive alternative.

d. It cannot detect partially occlusive thrombus.

II. Venous (upper and lower extremity) / Testing (20-25%)

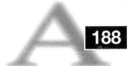
188

C. Duplex scanning is an accurate, noninvasive alternative.

The limitations of contrast venography include the risk of severe allergic reactions, relatively high expense, and patient discomfort.

▶ Rumwell C, McPharlin M: *Vascular Technology: An Illustrated Review,* 2nd edition. Pasadena, Davies Publishing, 2000, pp 200, 211.

Q 189

A nuclear medicine screening test that detects perfusion defects of the lungs is known as:

a.   bird's nest filter

b.   Greenfield filter

c.   VQ (ventilation quotient) scan

d.   ascending contrast venography

A **189**

C. VQ (ventilation quotient) scan.

190

A syndrome in which recurrent digital vasospasm occurs in response to cold exposure or stress is:

a. Raynaud's syndrome

b. Buerger's syndrome

c. thoracic outlet syndrome

d. Takayasu's syndrome

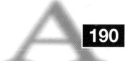

A. Raynaud's syndrome.

This vasospastic disorder most commonly occurs in women following exposure to cold or emotional stress. Classically, Raynaud's syndrome is characterized by profound skin pallor and numbness. Cyanosis occurs with warming of the digits, and then erythema follows accompanied by a burning pain.

▶ Rumwell C, McPharlin M: *Vascular Technology: An Illustrated Review,* 2nd edition. Pasadena, Davies Publishing, 2000, pp 35, 40, 81, 85, 226, 228.

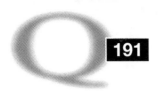

A disease involving thrombosis of the small or medium sized arteries of the extremities occurring predominantly in male smokers is:

a. Buerger's disease

b. Allen's disease

c. Raynaud's disease

d. thoracic outlet disease

191

A. Buerger's disease.

Q 192

An arteritis most commonly affecting the subclavian, renal, carotid, and ascending aorta in which more than 95% of patients are females is known as:

a. Takayasu's arteritis
b. temporal arteritis
c. polyarteritis nodosa
d. Kawasaki disease

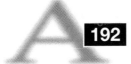

192

A. Takayasu's arteritis.

Takayasu's arteritis is a chronic inflammatory process that primarily affects the aorta and its major branches. The carotid bulb and proximal internal carotid artery are usually spared. More than 95% of affected patients are females in the second or third decade of life. Stenoses in these patients tend to be long, tapered, and smooth. These patients often have hypertension due to involvement of the renal arteries. Stroke is the presenting symptom in 14% of patients. Ultrasound findings include homogeneous segmental wall thickening, which has been termed the "macaroni" sign when viewed in transverse. This is usually associated with increased flow velocity through the affected area. In cerebrovascular involvement, homogeneous segmental wall thickening is usually limited to the common carotid and subclavian arteries. It is not uncommon to find occlusion of the common carotid artery with reversed flow in the ipsilateral external carotid artery to the patent ipsilateral internal carotid.

▶ Rumwell C, McPharlin M: *Vascular Technology: An Illustrated Review,* 2nd edition. Pasadena, Davies Publishing, 2000, p 39.
▶ Sun Y, Yip PK, Jeng JS, et al: Ultrasonographic study and long-term follow-up of Takayasu's arteritis. Stroke 27:2178–2182, 1996.

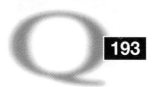
193

Hemorrhage within the layers of the arterial wall is known as:

a. ulceration
b. dissection
c. pseudoaneurysm
d. arteriovenous fistula

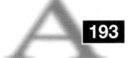

193

B. Dissection.

Dissection refers to hemorrhage within the wall of an artery. The hemorrhage may be localized within the media between the intima and media or it may involve the adventitia. When extravasated blood elevates the intima, an intimal flap results. Two lumens (a true and a false channel) can result, separated by an intimal flap. Usually there are multiple connections between the true and false lumen. Thrombosis of one lumen can occur, narrowing the artery. Dissections can occur spontaneously or as the result of trauma. Trauma may be either blunt or penetrating. Spontaneous dissections are related to systemic hypertension, fibromuscular dysplasia, cystic medial necrosis, Marfan's syndrome, or type IV Ehlers-Danlos syndrome. Sonographic findings include visualization of a mobile intimal flap or a long, smooth, and tapering stenosis suggesting thrombosis. Color Doppler can be useful in delineating flow within 2 distinct channels in the artery or demonstrating absence of flow in one lumen.

▶ Provenzale JM: Dissection of the internal carotid and vertebral arteries: imaging features. AJR 165:1099–1104, 1995.

Q **194**

A nonatherosclerotic, noninflammatory, occlusive, and aneurysmal disorder that primarily affects women and is referred to as a "string of beads" is:

a. Takayasu's disease

b. mycotic aneurysm

c. polyarteritis nodosa

d. fibromuscular dysplasia

A 194

D. Fibromuscular dysplasia.

Approximately 90% of cases of fibromuscular dysplasia occur in women. It most frequently affects the renal arteries, with carotid artery involvement being the next most common. Renal involvement may result in renovascular hypertension. Carotid involvement is most often benign, and most patients remain asymptomatic. Fewer than 10% of carotid lesions produce symptoms. One-half of patients with carotid involvement will have the disease in both carotid arteries. From 25% to 50% of patients with carotid fibromuscular dysplasia will have associated renal artery fibromuscular dysplasia. The vertebral artery is less frequently involved.

▶ Hurlbert SN, Krupski WC: Carotid artery disease in women. Semin Vasc Surg 8:268–276, 1995.

Q 195

A syndrome caused by swelling within the osteofascial compartments of the leg or arm resulting in decreased vascular perfusion is the:

a. compartment syndrome

b. Raynaud's syndrome

c. thoracic outlet syndrome

d. Marfan syndrome

A 195

A. Compartment syndrome.

This condition most commonly occurs after revascularization following prolonged ischemia, but may also develop due to external compression or bleeding within the compartment.

▶ Rumwell C, McPharlin M: *Vascular Technology: An Illustrated Review,* 2nd edition. Pasadena, Davies Publishing, 2000, p 111.

Q 196

Which syndrome results in medial displacement of the vessel due to compression by fibrous bands or the medial head of the gastrocnemius muscle?

a. thoracic outlet syndrome

b. popliteal entrapment syndrome

c. adductor canal compression syndrome

d. compartment syndrome

A 196

B. Popliteal entrapment syndrome.

This syndrome occurs when the artery is compressed by the medial head of the gastrocnemius muscle or fibrous bands. The popliteal artery is usually displaced medially. Popliteal entrapment syndrome is more common in young men and occurs bilaterally in up to one-third of cases. The trauma caused to the artery can result in the development of aneurysm, thrombosis, atherosclerosis, or embolic phenomena. Symptoms include intermittent claudication. Doppler findings include diminished or altered waveforms with knee extension, active plantar flexion, or passive dorsiflexion of the foot.

▶ Rumwell C, McPharlin M: *Vascular Technology: An Illustrated Review,* 2nd edition. Pasadena, Davies Publishing, 2000, pp 3, 111–112.

Q 197

Which of the following may be a source of emboli?

a. ulcerated atherosclerotic plaque

b. mural thrombus within an aneurysm

c. cardiac dysrhythmias

d. all of the above

A 197

D. All of the above.

An embolus is a plug—a foreign object—carried along in the bloodstream. It may be solid, liquid, or gaseous and may arise within the body or be introduced from without. Most commonly, an embolus is a fragment of thrombus or plaque that has dislodged from its origin and coursed distally in the blood stream before obstructing a small vessel. It may arise from ulcerative atherosclerotic plaque, mural thrombus in an aneurysm, or the heart.

▶ Rumwell C, McPharlin M: *Vascular Technology: An Illustrated Review,* 2nd edition. Pasadena, Davies Publishing, 2000, p 36.

Q 198

All of the following are risk factors for development of atherosclerotic disease **EXCEPT**:

a. diabetes mellitus

b. male sex

c. hypertension

d. underweight

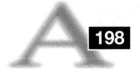

D. Underweight.

Dominant risk factors for the development of atherosclerotic disease include increasing age, male sex, cigarette smoking, diabetes mellitus, obesity, hyperlipidemia, hypertension, and positive family history for atherosclerotic disease.

▶ Parker BC, Bandyk DF, Mills JL, et al: Clinical evaluation of occlusive peripheral vascular disease. In Strandness DE, van Breda A (eds): *Vascular Diseases: Surgical and Interventional Therapy.* New York, Churchill Livingstone, 1994, pp 423–431.

Q 199

The most serious risk from femoropopliteal aneurysms is:

a. rupture

b. embolization

c. fistula

d. infection

A 199

B. Embolization.

The most serious risk from femoropopliteal aneurysms is lower limb ischemia from thrombosis or embolization. The most important features of these aneurysms are thrombus content and vessel tortuosity. These factors may result in sudden thrombosis and severe ischemia to the lower limb. The most serious risk of aortic aneurysms is rupture.

▶ Ballard DJ, Hallett JW: Natural history of aneurysms. In Strandness DE, van Breda A (eds): *Vascular Diseases: Surgical and Interventional Therapy.* New York, Churchill Livingstone, 1994, pp 565–569.

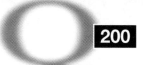

200

Cramping muscle pain which is induced by exercise and relieved by rest is termed:

a. claudication

b. bruit

c. rest pain

d. thrill

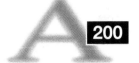

200

A. Claudication.

▶ Rumwell C, McPharlin M: *Vascular Technology: An Illustrated Review,* 2nd edition. Pasadena, Davies Publishing, 2000, pp 34, 59, 70, 111, 226, 248–249.

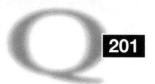

201

What severe symptom of decreased blood perfusion is aggravated by elevation, relieved by dependency, and often occurs when the patient goes to bed at night?

a. claudication

b. cyanosis

c. rest pain

d. postprandial pain

III. Peripheral Arterial / Signs and Symptoms (1–5%)

A 201

C. Rest pain.

▶ Rumwell C, McPharlin M: *Vascular Technology: An Illustrated Review,* 2nd edition. Pasadena, Davies Publishing, 2000, p 34.

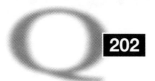

202

A smooth painful ulcer located on the dorsum of the foot is most likely a(n):

a. ischemic ulcer

b. stasis ulcer

c. lymphedema ulcer

d. neurotrophic ulcer

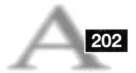

A. Ischemic ulcer.

Ischemic ulcers are most commonly located over pressure points such as the toe, heel, or dorsum of the foot. They may occur spontaneously or with trauma. Pain is often severe at night and is relieved by placing the extremity in a dependent position. The ulcer base is usually pale and the edge is definitive. The skin around it is atrophic or inflamed. Other trophic changes seen with arterial insufficiency include loss of hair on the affected extremity, shiny and smooth skin, thick brittle nails, and tapering of the toes or fingers. *Stasis ulcers* are caused by venous stasis in chronic venous insufficiency. They tend to occur over the medial distal third of the leg (gaiter zone). Pain is mild and is relieved by elevating the affected extremity. The ulcer edge appears uneven and the skin around the ulcer may show a brownish discoloration caused by hemosiderin deposits from the breakdown of red blood cells. *Neurotrophic ulcers* are associated with diabetes. They occur spontaneously and are located on the sole of the foot under calluses or on pressure points. They do not cause pain. The ulcer edge is definitive and the skin around it is callous.

▶ Rumwell C, McPharlin M: *Vascular Technology: An Illustrated Review,* 2nd edition. Pasadena, Davies Publishing, 2000, pp 39, 41, 185–186, 248.

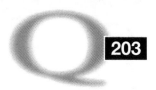

203

Which term describes a pale skin color due to insufficient blood flow?

a. pallor

b. cyanosis

c. rubor

d. rubella

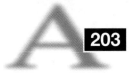

A. Pallor.

▶ Rumwell C, McPharlin M: *Vascular Technology: An Illustrated Review,* 2nd edition. Pasadena, Davies Publishing, 2000, pp 35, 39–40, 90, 185.

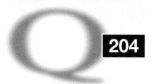

204

Which of the following is **NOT** true regarding bruits?

a. A bruit is a low-frequency sound heard on auscultation.

b. A prominent bruit will be heard over an arterial occlusion.

c. The absence of a bruit cannot rule out disease.

d. A bruit persisting through diastole is usually associated with severe stenosis.

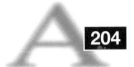

204

B. This statement—"a prominent bruit will be heard over an arterial occlusion"—is NOT true.

A bruit is a vibratory reaction in the tissue distal to a stenosis. It will not be present with complete occlusion or trickle flow in high-grade stenosis.

▶ Rumwell C, McPharlin M: *Vascular Technology: An Illustrated Review,* 2nd edition. Pasadena, Davies Publishing, 2000, pp 22, 42, 86, 106, 135, 255, 306–307.

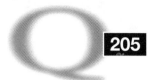

205

A patient presents to the vascular lab with the history of recent brachial artery catheterization and a palpable thrill over the brachial artery. Which diagnosis is most likely?

a. complete thrombosis of the brachial artery

b. deep venous thrombosis of the brachial vein

c. hematoma surrounding the brachial artery

d. arteriovenous fistula involving the brachial artery and vein

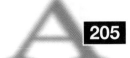

205

D. Arteriovenous fistula of the brachial artery and vein.

A vascular *thrill* is a palpable vibration over an artery. It indicates a high-flow state with turbulence and is commonly felt over a fistula site. In this case, the patient reports a recent brachial artery catheterization. Complications of arterial catheterization include arteriovenous fistula, pseudoaneurysm, hematoma, and thrombosis. Of these, only the fistula and possibly the pseudoaneurysms will produce a palpable thrill.

▶ Rumwell C, McPharlin M: *Vascular Technology: An Illustrated Review,* 2nd edition. Pasadena, Davies Publishing, 2000, pp 42, 86.

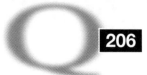

206

The best way for a vascular technologist to palpate a pulse is to:

a. place his thumb over the pulse site
b. place the back of his hand over the pulse site
c. place his fingertips over the pulse site
d. push hard over the pulse site with both hands

A 206

C. Place his fingertips over the pulse site.

When the thumb is used to palpate a pulse, the examiner cannot determine if the origin of the pulse is from the patient or himself. The best way to palpate a pulse is to place your fingertips over the pulse site.

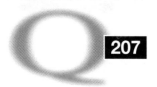

207

Palpation of a pulse found in the groove behind the medial malleolus of the ankle corresponds to the:

a. posterior tibial artery
b. anterior tibial artery
c. peroneal artery
d. plantar artery

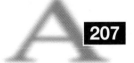

A. Posterior tibial artery.

▶ Fahey VA, White SA: Physical assessment of the vascular system. In Fahey VA (ed): *Vascular Nursing*. Philadelphia, Saunders, 1988, pp 51–68.

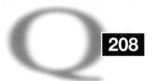

208

The presence of a bruit indicates:

a. arterial stenosis proximal to the point of auscultation
b. arterial occlusion directly beneath the point of auscultation
c. the absence of arterial disease
d. venous thrombosis

A 208

A. Arterial stenosis proximal to the point of auscultation.

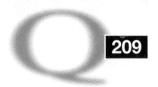

209

A patient with a history of tibial artery surgical repair now presents with foot drop, muscle necrosis, and severe pain. What diagnosis is suspected?

a. arteriovenous fistula

b. pseudoaneurysm

c. compartment syndrome

d. Raynaud's syndrome

A 209

C. Compartment syndrome.

Q 210

What vein is most commonly used in the lower extremity as a reversed vein bypass graft?

a. greater saphenous vein

b. cephalic vein

c. femoral vein

d. lesser saphenous vein

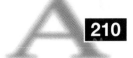

210

A. Greater saphenous vein.

The greater saphenous vein (GSV) is the vein of choice for reversed vein grafts in the lower extremity. If the GSV is unavailable, the cephalic or brachial veins may be used.

▶ Rumwell C, McPharlin M: *Vascular Technology: An Illustrated Review,* 2nd edition. Pasadena, Davies Publishing, 2000, pp 93–94, 116–117.

▶ Ridgway DP: *Introduction to Vascular Scanning: A Guide for the Complete Beginner,* 2nd edition. Pasadena, Davies Publishing, 1999, pp 160–161.

211

Which bypass graft has a size discrepancy between the graft and the native artery at both the proximal and distal anastomotic sites?

a. in situ vein graft

b. reversed vein graft

c. synthetic graft

d. Greenfield graft

A 211

B. Reversed vein graft.

In a reversed vein graft, the vein (usually the greater saphenous vein) is surgically lifted from its bed and reversed before being attached to the normal portion of the native artery. An advantage of this technique is that the venous valves are oriented in the direction of blood flow. Additionally, all vein branches are easily ligated since the entire vein has been exposed during surgery. A disadvantage is the caliber discrepancy between the graft and the native artery at both anastomotic sites. This occurs because the saphenous vein is normally larger in the thigh and smaller at the ankle. Reversing the vein results in the smaller end being connected to the largest part of the native artery and the larger end being connected to the smallest part of the native artery.

▶ Rumwell C, McPharlin M: *Vascular Technology: An Illustrated Review,* 2nd edition. Pasadena, Davies Publishing, 2000, pp 93–96.
▶ Polak JF: Arterial sonography: efficacy for the diagnosis of arterial disease of the lower extremity. AJR 161:235–243, 1993.

212

Which bypass graft would most likely be seen in a patient with bilateral common iliac artery obstruction?

a. femoral to posterior tibial artery
b. femoral to femoral
c. femoral to popliteal
d. aortobifemoral

A 212

D. Aortobifemoral.

213

What is the most common form of nonsurgical intervention for focal atherosclerotic disease in the lower extremity?

a. atherectomy

b. thrombectomy

c. angioplasty

d. endarterectomy

A 213

C. Angioplasty.

Also known as balloon angioplasty (percutaneous transluminal angioplasty [PTA]), angioplasty is performed by inserting a balloon-tipped catheter into an artery, positioning the tip of the catheter within the stenotic segment to be dilated, and slowly inflating the balloon, which pushes the plaque against the vessel wall and enlarges the vessel lumen to a normal or nearly normal diameter.

▶ Rumwell C, McPharlin M: *Vascular Technology: An Illustrated Review,* 2nd edition. Pasadena, Davies Publishing, 2000, p 118.

Q 214

A complication following femoral artery catheterization in which a characteristic to-and-fro Doppler waveform is seen within a tract leading to a perivascular hematoma is termed a(n):

a. arteriovenous fistula

b. pseudoaneurysm

c. occlusion

d. mycotic aneurysm

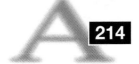

B. Pseudoaneurysm.

Pseudoaneurysms occur when a puncture site fails to close and blood escapes into the surrounding tissue forming a perivascular hematoma. Color and spectral Doppler can be used to confirm the vascular nature of the mass and to identify the tract or neck leading from the native vessel to the pseudoaneurysm. The Doppler waveform obtained within the pseudoaneurysm will be turbulent. The Doppler waveform obtained from the neck will show a classic to-and-fro flow pattern with high velocities.

▶ Rumwell C, McPharlin M: *Vascular Technology: An Illustrated Review,* 2nd edition. Pasadena, Davies Publishing, 2000, pp 119–120.
▶ Hertz SM, Brener BJ: Ultrasound-guided pseudoaneurysm compression: efficacy after coronary stenting and angioplasty. J Vasc Surg 26:913–918, 1997.

Q 215

Which of the following is a late complication of extremity bypass grafts?

a. pseudoaneurysm
b. arteriovenous fistula
c. hematoma
d. intimal hyperplasia

215

D. Intimal hyperplasia.

Hematomas and pseudoaneurysms associated with extremity bypass grafts are usually seen in the immediate postoperative period. Arteriovenous fistulas occur because of failure to ligate a vein branch and are typically discovered as an early complication following surgery. Arteriovenous fistulas also may spontaneously open or close with the changing hemodynamics of the graft. Intimal hyperplasia is a late complication of bypass grafts resulting from the accumulation of smooth muscle cells and matrix forming a fibrous thickening in the graft. This can occur either focally or diffusely and lead to stenosis. It tends to occur at the anastomotic sites, venous valve sites, and clamp sites.

▶ Hertz SM, Brener BJ: Ultrasound-guided pseudoaneurysm compression: efficacy after coronary stenting and angioplasty. J Vasc Surg 26:913–918, 1997.

▶ Polak JF: Arterial sonography: efficacy for the diagnosis of arterial disease of the lower extremity. AJR 161:235–243, 1993.

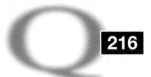

216

A technique in which atherosclerotic plaque is mechanically removed by cutting or pulverizing it and then extracted by suction or downstream embolization is termed:

a. atherectomy
b. thrombectomy
c. angioplasty
d. endarterectomy

A **216**

A. Atherectomy.

▶ Rumwell C, McPharlin M: *Vascular Technology: An Illustrated Review,* 2nd edition. Pasadena, Davies Publishing, 2000, pp 118–119.

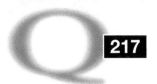

217

What quantitative index is calculated by dividing the peak-to-peak frequency difference by the mean frequency?

a. resistive index
b. volume index
c. pulsatility index
d. acceleration index

A 217

C. Pulsatility index.

▶ Rumwell C, McPharlin M: *Vascular Technology: An Illustrated Review,* 2nd edition. Pasadena, Davies Publishing, 2000, p 51.

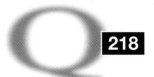

218

What measurement helps in differentiation of inflow versus outflow disease by measuring the time between the onset of systole to the maximum systolic peak?

a. resistive index

b. acceleration time

c. volume flow

d. A/B ratio

A **218**

B. Acceleration time.

▶ Rumwell C, McPharlin M: *Vascular Technology: An Illustrated Review,* 2nd edition. Pasadena, Davies Publishing, 2000, p 103.

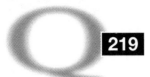

219

Which method of Doppler Display exhibits a grayscale trace representing the entire range of reflected frequency shifts from the location of the sample volume?

a. analog waveform

b. power Doppler

c. spectral analysis

d. color flow

DAVIES
Registry Reviews & Study Aids

A 219

C. Spectral analysis.

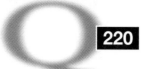

Q 220

A high-pitched signal heard on audible Doppler analysis always indicates:

a. the presence of high-velocity flow

b. high-frequency shifts

c. the presence of a stenosis

d. a vessel kink

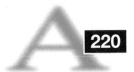

B. High-frequency shifts.

A high-frequency shift produces a higher-pitched signal. The magnitude of the Doppler frequency shift is determined not only by the speed of the flow, but also by the angle at which the Doppler beam intersects the flow (the Doppler "look" angle), and the Doppler frequency. Since the Doppler frequency is constant during a given Doppler sampling, the two factors that can be responsible for increased pitch (frequency) are high blood flow velocity and decreased angle of incidence. This fact is demonstrated by the Doppler equation: Frequency shift = 2 f V cosθ ÷ c, where f = operating frequency of the Doppler transducer, V = velocity of blood flow, cosθ = cosine of Doppler "look" angle, c = speed of ultrasound in soft tissue (i.e., 1540 m/sec).

▶ Rumwell C, McPharlin M: *Vascular Technology: An Illustrated Review,* 2nd edition. Pasadena, Davies Publishing, 2000, pp 32, 44–45, 54, 62, 86.

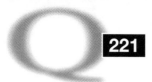

221

When taking ankle pressures, the patient should be:

a. sitting

b. standing

c. supine

d. reverse Trendelenburg

A 221

C. Supine.

Ankle pressures should be obtained with the patient supine and in a resting state.

▶ Rumwell C, McPharlin M: *Vascular Technology: An Illustrated Review,* 2nd edition. Pasadena, Davies Publishing, 2000, p 53.

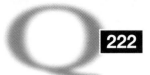

222

What is an appropriately sized cuff for obtaining pressures in the fingers?

a. 0.5–1 cm

b. 2–2.5 cm

c. 3 cm

d. 5 cm

A 222

B. 2.0–2.5 cm.

▶ Rumwell C, McPharlin M: *Vascular Technology: An Illustrated Review,* 2nd edition. Pasadena, Davies Publishing, 2000, p 79.

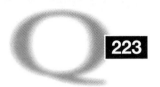

223

Which of the following correctly describes an advantage of pulsed wave (PW) Doppler over continuous wave (CW) Doppler?

a. PW Doppler does not exhibit aliasing.

b. PW Doppler is more accurate in measuring high velocities.

c. PW Doppler is more accurate in measuring low velocities.

d. Echoes can be received from a specific location with PW Doppler.

D. Echoes can be received from a specific location with PW Doppler.

This is termed range-gating. Since the speed of sound in tissue is known (1540 m/s), the round-trip time to a specific depth (sample volume location) is easily determined. The system sends a pulse and then waits the calculated time to receive echoes only from the desired depth. This is not possible with CW Doppler, in which echoes are continually received from all moving interfaces encountered in the path of the beam.

Q **224**

An acceleration time of less than 133 msec obtained in the femoral artery suggests:

a. proximal iliac artery stenosis

b. distal femoral artery occlusion

c. pseudoaneurysm of the femoral artery

d. the absence of significant iliac artery disease

A 224

D. The absence of significant iliac artery disease.

A rapid upstroke in systole results in a short acceleration time. This pattern is consistent with normal inflow. A delayed upstroke occurs with significant inflow disease (stenosis proximal to the site of sampling).

▶ Rumwell C, McPharlin M: *Vascular Technology: An Illustrated Review,* 2nd edition. Pasadena, Davies Publishing, 2000, pp 51–52, 103.

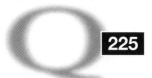

225

A disease in which segmental pressure studies may show falsely elevated Doppler pressures due to arterial wall calcification is:

a. diabetes mellitus

b. Takayasu's arteritis

c. Marfan's syndrome

d. Raynaud's syndrome

A 225

A. Diabetes mellitus.

The vessels of patients with diabetes may be incompressible because of arterial wall calcification, a condition that leads to falsely elevated pressures.

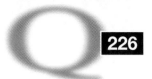

226

The ankle/brachial index is calculated by dividing the ankle pressure by:

a. the right brachial pressure

b. the left brachial pressure

c. the highest of the two brachial pressures

d. the lowest of the two brachial pressures

A 226

C. The highest of the two brachial pressures.

▶ Rumwell C, McPharlin M: *Vascular Technology: An Illustrated Review,* 2nd edition. Pasadena, Davies Publishing, 2000, p 56.

Q 227

Using the four-cuff technique for segmental pressures, normal high thigh pressures are _____ the brachial pressure.

a. equal to
b. at least 30 mmHg greater than
c. at least 30 mmHg less than
d. not compared to

A 227

B. At least 30 mmHg greater than.

Using the four-cuff technique for segmental pressures, the high thigh cuff is small in diameter compared to the limb. This results in an artifactually elevated pressure at the high-thigh site. Therefore, normal pressures obtained at the high-thigh level are at least 30 mmHg greater than the highest brachial pressure.

▶ Rumwell C, McPharlin M: *Vascular Technology: An Illustrated Review,* 2nd edition. Pasadena, Davies Publishing, 2000, p 57.

Q 228

In a normal study, the ankle systolic pressure should be:

a. less than the highest brachial blood pressure
b. the same or greater than the highest brachial blood pressure
c. equal to the lowest brachial blood pressure
d. less than the right brachial blood pressure

A 228

B. The same or greater than the highest brachial blood pressure.

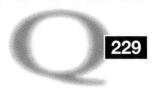

229

When measuring segmental pressures, gradients of 20–30 mmHg between corresponding segments of the legs indicates:

a. disease at or above the level in the leg with lower pressure
b. disease below the level in the leg with higher pressure
c. disease above the level in the leg with higher pressure
d. no significant disease

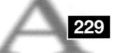
A. Disease at or above the level in the leg with lower pressure.

In addition to pressure gradients between segments on a single limb, horizontal gradients between two limbs at the same level indicate obstructive disease at or above the level in the leg with the lower pressure.

▶ Rumwell C, McPharlin M: *Vascular Technology: An Illustrated Review,* 2nd edition. Pasadena, Davies Publishing, 2000, p 57.

230

Following exercise, what is a normal response for ankle pressures in comparison with resting values?

a. no change

b. decrease

c. increase

d. gradual decrease over 5 minutes

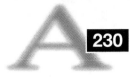

C. Increase.

In a patient without obstructive disease, ankle pressures will increase following exercise. In the presence of arterial obstructive disease, the ankle pressure will decrease immediately after exercise.

▶ Rumwell C, McPharlin M: *Vascular Technology: An Illustrated Review,* 2nd edition. Pasadena, Davies Publishing, 2000, p 60.

Q 231

A 57-year-old male presented to the vascular lab for lower extremity arterial testing. Exercise testing was stopped due to symptoms of claudication. Postexercise ankle pressures measured slightly above resting ankle pressures. What is suspected in this patient?

a. a nonvascular cause of leg pain

b. occlusion or stenosis at a single level

c. multilevel arterial disease

d. isolated iliac artery occlusion

A **231**

A. A nonvascular cause of leg pain.

If a patient must stop exercising because of leg pain but shows normal ankle pressures, a nonvascular cause of leg pain should be considered.

▶ Rumwell C, McPharlin M: *Vascular Technology: An Illustrated Review,* 2nd edition. Pasadena, Davies Publishing, 2000, pp 59–60.

Q 232

An aneurysm resulting from infection is known as:

a. fusiform

b. saccular

c. mycotic

d. ectatic

DAVIES
Registry Reviews & Study Aids

A 232

C. Mycotic.

Q 233

A volume plethysmographic waveform with a normal amplitude, rounded peak, and an absent dicrotic wave is most likely indicative of:

a. normal arterial inflow

b. arterial disease proximal to the level of tracing

c. arterial disease distal to the level of tracing

d. arterial occlusion at the level of the tracing

A 233

B. Arterial disease proximal to the level of tracing.

A volume plethysmographic waveform with a flattened systolic peak and absent dicrotic notch is moderately abnormal and always reflects arterial disease proximal to the level of the tracing. Other signs of moderate abnormality include a decrease in the upslope and downslope time that is nearly equal between upslope and downslope.

▶ Rumwell C, McPharlin M: *Vascular Technology: An Illustrated Review,* 2nd edition. Pasadena, Davies Publishing, 2000, pp 74–75.

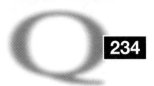

234

To obtain digital pressures of the toes, how should the patient be positioned?

a. supine

b. decubitus

c. Trendelenburg

d. standing

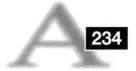

234

A. Supine.

The patient should be in a supine position while the examiner obtains toe pressures. The head can be elevated 10–20 degrees.

▶ Rumwell C, McPharlin M: *Vascular Technology: An Illustrated Review,* 2nd edition. Pasadena, Davies Publishing, 2000, p 77.

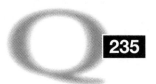

235

A type of plethysmography that detects cutaneous blood flow by sending infrared light into the tissue is termed:

a. strain gauge plethysmography

b. volume plethysmography

c. impedance plethysmography

d. photoplethysmography

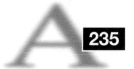

D. Photoplethysmography.

Photoplethysmography detects cutaneous blood flow by sending infrared light into the tissue with a light-emitting diode. A photodetector receives and measures the reflected infrared light.

▶ Rumwell C, McPharlin M: *Vascular Technology: An Illustrated Review,* 2nd edition. Pasadena, Davies Publishing, 2000, pp 70–77.

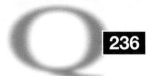

236

Following cessation of exercise in a normal individual, how long does it take for lower extremity blood flow to return to resting values?

a. 1–5 minutes

b. 5–10 minutes

c. 10–15 minutes

d. as long as 30 minutes

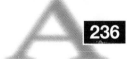

A. 1 to 5 minutes.

▶ Strandness DE, Zierler RE: Exercise ankle pressure measurements in arterial disease. In Bernstein EF (ed): *Noninvasive Diagnostic Techniques in Vascular Disease.* St. Louis, Mosby, 1985, pp 575–583.

Q 237

The best method for evaluation of suspected popliteal aneurysm is:

a. pulse volume recording

b. segmental pressures

c. continuous-wave Doppler

d. duplex ultrasound

237

D. Duplex ultrasound.

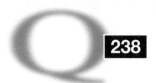

238

A 59-year-old female presents gradual onset of edema beginning at the dorsum of the foot and proceeding proximally. The swelling is not relieved by leg elevation. These symptoms most closely relate to which condition?

a. lymphedema

b. superficial venous thrombosis

c. arterial ischemia

d. embolization

238

A. Lymphedema.

Lymphedema may be congenital or acquired. Acquired lymphedema usually involves the entire lower extremity and may be associated with a minor event such as an insect bite, ankle sprain, or cutaneous infection. The edema is usually not associated with other symptoms. It begins at the dorsum of the foot and proceeds proximally. There is no cutaneous pigmentation, dermatitis, or ulceration as in venous edema, although long-term cases may show hyperkeratosis of the skin. Lymphedema can be further differentiated from venous edema because venous edema will improve quickly with leg elevation but lymphedema will not.

▶ Dixon MB, Bergan JJ: Lymphedema. In Fahey VA (ed): *Vascular Nursing.* Philadelphia, Saunders, 1988, pp 33–47.

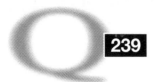

239

The segmental pressure measurements listed below were obtained from a 67-year-old male with symptoms of claudication.

Right	Segment	Left
160 mmHg	brachial	172 mmHg
189 mmHg	high thigh	150 mmHg
161 mmHg	above knee	126 mmHg
157 mmHg	below knee	104 mmHg
118 mmHg	ankle	84 mmHg

What values are used to determine the ABI?

a. right 118/160, left 84/172

b. right 118/172, left 84/172

c. right 118/160, left 84/160

d. right 118/172, left 84/160

DAVIES
Registry Reviews & Study Aids

A 239

B. Right 118/172, left 84/172.

The ABIs are right ABI = 0.68 and left ABI = 0.48.

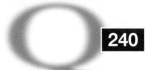

240

A 72-year-old female is referred to the vascular lab for evaluation of right lower extremity claudication. Brachial blood pressures are 135 mmHg (bilateral) and ankle pressures are 300 mmHg. This is most likely related to:

a. severe hypertension

b. cuff artifact due to improper size

c. misalignment of cuff on the extremity

d. incompressible arteries due to arterial calcification

A **240**

D. Incompressible arteries due to arterial calcification.

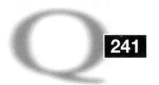

241

A 58-year-old male presents to the vascular lab with an abdominal bruit and bilateral weak lower extremity pulses. Review the segmental pressures below and determine the level of disease.

Right	Segment	Left
155 mmHg	brachial	148 mmHg
101 mmHg	high thigh	100 mmHg
98 mmHg	above knee	98 mmHg
89 mmHg	below knee	89 mmHg
87 mmHg	ankle	88 mmHg

a. right deep femoral artery, left popliteal

b. aortoiliac disease

c. right superficial femoral artery obstruction, left popliteal artery obstruction

d. bilateral trifurcation disease

III. Peripheral Arterial / Testing (upper and lower extremity) (15–20%)

A 241

B. Aortoiliac disease.

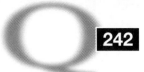

242

Determine the ABIs from the above segmental pressure study.

a. right 0.56, left 0.56
b. right 0.56, left 0.59
c. right 0.59, left 0.56
d. right 1.78, left 1.68

484

A 242

A. Right 0.56, left 0.56.

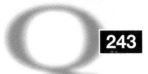

243

A test used to detect arterial patency of the palmar arch is termed:

a. strain gauge plethysmography

b. reactive hyperemia

c. thoracic outlet evaluation

d. Allen's test

A **243**

D. Allen's test.

Q 244

A Doppler tracing performed at the medial malleolus is obtained from what artery?

a. posterior tibial
b. dorsalis pedis
c. peroneal
d. anterior tibial

A 244

A. Posterior tibial.

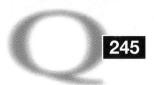

245

Which of the following can result in a loss of the triphasic waveform in the popliteal artery?

a. distal vasodilatation

b. proximal occlusion

c. postexercise

d. all of the above

A 245

D. All of the above.

Q 246

A dampened waveform demonstrating a delayed acceleration time is obtained in the common femoral artery. This is most likely due to which of the following?

a. inflow disease
b. distal occlusion
c. pseudoaneurysm
d. postexercise

A **246**

A. Inflow disease.

▶ Rumwell C, McPharlin M: *Vascular Technology: An Illustrated Review,* 2nd edition. Pasadena, Davies Publishing, 2000, pp 51–52.

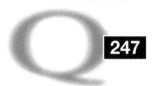

247

To obtain segmental pressures of the lower extremity, the patient should be positioned:

a. reverse Trendelenburg
b. Trendelenburg
c. supine with the extremities at the same level as the heart
d. supine with the extremities below the level of the heart

A 247

C. Supine with the extremities at the same level as the heart.

▶ Rumwell C, McPharlin M: *Vascular Technology: An Illustrated Review,* 2nd edition. Pasadena, Davies Publishing, 2000, p 53.

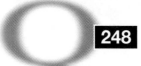

248

Which ABI is indicative of rest pain?

a. > 1.0

b. 0.9–1.0

c. 0.5–0.9

d. < 0.5

III. Peripheral Arterial / Testing (upper and lower extremity) (15–20%)

248

D. < 0.5.

249

Evaluate the segmental pressures presented below. The horizontal difference of 28 mmHg at the level below the knee is most likely due to:

Right	Segment	Left
150 mmHg	brachial	151 mmHg
189 mmHg	high thigh	192 mmHg
178 mmHg	above knee	173 mmHg
134 mmHg	below knee	162 mmHg
97 mmHg	ankle	152 mmHg

a. cuff artifact

b. right popliteal and tibial vessel disease

c. left femoral artery disease

d. right inflow disease

A 249

B. Right popliteal and tibial vessel disease.

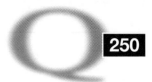

250

A toe pressure of 30 mmHg or less indicates:

a. a good chance of healing for foot or toe ulcer
b. poor chance of healing for foot or toe ulcer
c. arterial calcification due to diabetes
d. normality

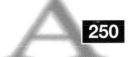

250

B. Poor chance of healing for foot or toe ulcer.

Great toe pressures are especially useful in diabetic patients in whom ankle pressures are unreliable because of arterial calcification. The normal toe pressure is 60 mmHg. When toe pressures are 30 mmHg or less, foot or toe ulcerations are unlikely to heal.

▶ Rumwell C, McPharlin M: *Vascular Technology: An Illustrated Review,* 2nd edition. Pasadena, Davies Publishing, 2000, p 58.

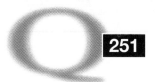

251

Contraindications for treadmill stress testing include all of the following **EXCEPT**:

a. history of cardiac problems
b. history of stroke
c. history of claudication
d. shortness of breath

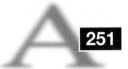

C. History of claudication.

Exercise testing is used to help differentiate between true claudication and neurogenic claudication and to help determine the presence or absence of collaterals. It is indicated when resting measurements are not grossly abnormal and/or symptoms do not correlate with the resting measurements. Contraindications to exercise stress testing include shortness of breath, hypertension, cardiac problems, stroke, and walking problems.

▶ Rumwell C, McPharlin M: *Vascular Technology: An Illustrated Review,* 2nd edition. Pasadena, Davies Publishing, 2000, p 59.

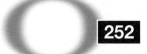

252

A stenosis of the superficial femoral artery showed a peak systolic velocity of 180 cm/sec and a prestenotic velocity of 85 cm/sec. What percentage diameter stenosis is suggested by these values?

a. ≥25%

b. ≥50%

c. ≥75%

d. ≥90%

III. Peripheral Arterial / Testing (upper and lower extremity) (15–20%)

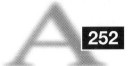

252

B. ≥50%.

In duplex evaluation of the lower extremity arterial circulation, a ratio is calculated between the prestenotic systolic velocity and the peak systolic velocity within the stenosis. A 2:1 ratio suggests a greater than 50% diameter stenosis, and a 4:1 ratio suggests a greater than 75% diameter stenosis.

▶ Rumwell C, McPharlin M: *Vascular Technology: An Illustrated Review,* 2nd edition. Pasadena, Davies Publishing, 2000, pp 94–95.

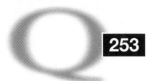

253

In performing reactive hyperemia testing, the blood pressure cuffs are inflated to suprasystolic pressure levels for:

a. 45 seconds

b. 1–2 minute

c. 8 minutes

d. 3–5 minutes

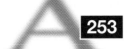

D. 3–5 minutes.

Reactive hyperemia testing is an alternative method to exercise testing for stressing the peripheral arterial system. The blood pressure cuff is inflated above the highest brachial blood pressure for 3–5 minutes. This test is very uncomfortable for the patient. Ischemia and vasodilatation occur distal to the cuff. Once the cuff is released, the changes in ankle pressure are similar to those obtained after exercise, although a transient decrease in pressure of 17–34% may be seen in normal limbs with reactive hyperemia.

▶ Rumwell C, McPharlin M: *Vascular Technology: An Illustrated Review,* 2nd edition. Pasadena, Davies Publishing, 2000, p 61.

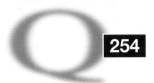

254

Retrograde flow in the native artery at the site of distal anastomosis of a lower extremity bypass graft is:

a. a normal finding

b. an early indication of graft failure

c. indicative of arteriovenous fistula

d. diagnostic of distal occlusive disease

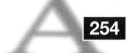

A. A normal finding.

Blood flow always courses in a direction from high pressure to low pressure. In this case, there is higher pressure within the normal graft and lower pressure within the native artery. This commonly results in some blood coursing up (retrograde) the native artery at the site of the distal anastomosis. This retrograde flow perfuses tissue above the level of the anastomotic site and provides additional benefit to the patient.

▶ Rumwell C, McPharlin M: *Vascular Technology: An Illustrated Review,* 2nd edition. Pasadena, Davies Publishing, 2000, p 94.

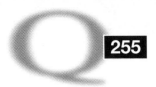

Q 255

Which statement is **NOT** true regarding arteriography?

a. requires an intraarterial injection

b. gives functional information regarding vascular system

c. gives anatomic information regarding vascular system

d. employs a liquid contrast agent to image arterial lumen

A **255**

B. This statement—"gives functional information regarding vascular system"—is NOT true.

Arteriography gives anatomic but not functional (physiologic) information.

▶ Rumwell C, McPharlin M: *Vascular Technology: An Illustrated Review,* 2nd edition. Pasadena, Davies Publishing, 2000, p 115.

Q 256

Vasospasm is demonstrated arteriographically as:

a. a vibrating artery
b. an appearance described as a "string of beads"
c. a severe narrowing of the arterial lumen
d. vasospasm cannot be detected arteriographically

A 256

C. A severe narrowing of the arterial lumen.

▶ Rumwell C, McPharlin M: *Vascular Technology: An Illustrated Review,* 2nd edition. Pasadena, Davies Publishing, 2000, p 115.

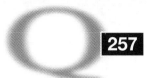

257

Arteriography is contraindicated in a patient with which condition?

a. diabetic

b. renal failure

c. malignancy

d. vascular disease

A 257

B. Renal failure.

▶ Rumwell C, McPharlin M: *Vascular Technology: An Illustrated Review,* 2nd edition. Pasadena, Davies Publishing, 2000, p 116.

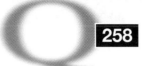

258

The most common cause of portal hypertension in the United States is:

a. schistosomiasis

b. cirrhosis

c. hyperlipedemia

d. hypertension

A 258

B. Cirrhosis.

259

You have received a request to evaluate blood flow within the splanchnic arteries. Which of the following groups of blood vessels should you examine?

a. celiac artery, superior mesenteric artery, inferior mesenteric artery

b. main portal vein, right portal vein, left portal vein

c. right and left renal arteries and veins

d. right and left common iliac and external iliac arteries

A 259

A. Celiac artery, superior mesenteric artery, inferior mesenteric artery.

The splanchnic arteries are the vessels that supply blood to the gut. These primarily are the celiac artery, superior mesenteric artery (SMA), and inferior mesenteric artery (IMA). Stenosis or occlusion involving these vessels can result in chronic ischemia of the bowel, known as *mesenteric ischemia*.

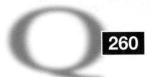

260

You are performing a Doppler exam on a patient with suspected renovascular hypertension. Which diagnostic parameter is the best indicator of renovascular disease?

a. pulsatility index

b. A/B ratio

c. renal/aortic ratio

d. systolic/diastolic ratio

A 260

C. Renal/aortic ratio.

Renovascular hypertension is caused by renal artery stenosis. Stenosis of the renal artery can be determined by obtaining a renal/aortic ratio (RAR). This is a ratio of the highest velocity obtained in the renal artery to the normal velocity of the aorta obtained at the level of the renal artery origins. A ratio of ≥ 3.5 is considered by most to indicate a significant renal artery stenosis. This would mean that the velocity in the renal artery is 3.5 times faster than the velocity in the aorta.

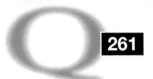

261

What abdominal vessel is most commonly compromised by compression of the median arcuate ligament of the diaphragm?

a. inferior vena cava

b. left gastric artery

c. superior mesenteric artery

d. celiac artery

A 261

D. Celiac artery

The median arcuate ligament of the diaphragm crosses the anterior aspect of the aorta slightly above (i.e., superior to) the celiac trunk. In some patients, during expiration, this anatomic situation can lead to compression of the celiac artery and high velocities. The abnormally high velocities are present during expiration but return to normal during inspiration. These patients may present with an abdominal bruit.

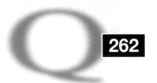

262

Which of the following is **NOT** a common feature of renal allograft rejection?

a. increased allograft size

b. increased cortical echogenicity

c. decreased flow resistance in parenchymal arteries

d. increased prominence of the renal pyramids

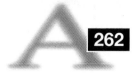

262

C. Decreased flow resistance in parenchymal arteries.

In renal allograft rejection the flow resistance in the parenchymal arteries tends to increase. This will be manifested as a decrease in diastolic flow. Normal flow in the parenchymal arteries of a renal allograft is low resistance with forward flow throughout the cardiac cycle. A decrease, absence, or reversal of flow in diastole is indicative of rejection.

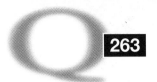

263

Which of the following would be most likely to occur as a result of increased portal venous pressure in a patient with portal hypertension?

a.   cavernous transformation

b.   aortic dissection

c.   hepatic artery aneurysm

d.   enlarged coronary vein

A 263

D. Enlarged coronary vein.

The coronary vein normally drains into the splenic vein. With portal hypertension, the increased portal venous pressure decreases flow into the portal system. Consequently, vessels that normally drain into the portal system become enlarged and often find alternate routes of flow. The coronary vein may reverse its flow direction and feed into esophageal varices. These can break down, causing life-threatening bleeding episodes. Cavernous transformation may occur in patients with portal hypertension, but only in the presence of portal vein thrombosis and recanalization. Cavernous transformation of the portal vein most commonly occurs when the liver is normal. Most patients with portal hypertension have underlying liver cirrhosis. Aortic dissection and hepatic artery aneurysm are not associated with portal hypertension.

Q 264

What is the most common location of atherosclerotic disease of the renal artery?

a. proximal
b. mid
c. distal
d. intrarenal

A 264

A. Proximal

Atherosclerotic disease tends to affect the bifurcations of arteries. The renal artery is most commonly affected at its origin from the aorta. This is considered to be the proximal portion of the vessel. Fibromuscular disease more commonly affects the mid to distal aspect of the renal artery.

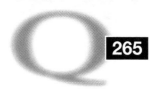

265

You are performing a Doppler study on a patient with fibromuscular dysplasia. Which of the following conditions is most commonly associated with this abnormality?

a. renovascular hypertension

b. portal hypertension

c. mesenteric ischemia

d. Budd-Chiari syndrome

A **265**

A. Renovascular hypertension.

Fibromuscular hyperplasia is a condition in which the artery has a series of small dilatations and narrowings that create the angiographic appearance of a string of beads or pearls. In contrast to atherosclerosis, fibromuscular hyperplasia tends to affect younger individuals and is more common in women than men. It can affect the renal arteries and tends to be located in the mid to distal end of the vessel. The splanchnic vessels are uncommonly affected.

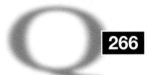

266

A patient presents to the vascular lab with an abdominal bruit, weight loss, and postprandial pain. Obstruction of which vessel is most likely responsible for these symptoms?

a. renal arteries

b. portal vein

c. superior mesenteric artery

d. splenic vein

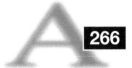

A 266

C. Superior mesenteric artery.

Chronic mesenteric ischemia may result from obstruction of the arteries that supply the gut. The primary vessel supplying the intestine is the superior mesenteric artery. The inferior mesenteric artery and celiac trunk may also contribute. Symptoms usually do not occur unless 2 of these 3 arteries are obstructed. A rich collateral network exists between these three vessels, making chronic mesenteric ischemia a rare disorder.

▶ Baxter BT, Pearce WH: Diagnosis and surgical management of chronic mesenteric ischemia. In Strandness DE, van Breda A (eds): *Vascular Diseases: Surgical and Interventional Therapy.* New York, Churchill Livingstone, 1994, pp 795–802.

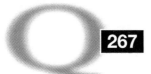

Q 267

An enlarged coronary vein with retrograde flow is a sign of:

a. inferior vena cava thrombus

b. renal vein thrombus

c. iliac vein thrombus

d. portal hypertension

A 267

D. Portal hypertension.

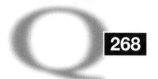

268

This Doppler waveform was obtained from a segmental artery within the kidney in a patient with severe hypertension. Which diagnosis is most likely?

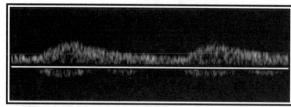

a. presence of parenchymal renal disease

b. presence of ipsilateral main renal artery stenosis

c. ipsilateral renal vein thrombosis

d. renal failure

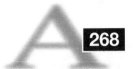

268

B. Presence of ipsilateral main renal artery stenosis.

The delayed systolic upstroke and absence of early systolic peak in the waveform of this segmental renal artery indicates proximal stenosis of greater than 60 percent in the main renal artery. This waveform shape is termed tardus and parvus.

Stavros T, Harshfield D: Renal Doppler, renal artery stenosis, and renovascular hypertension: direct and indirect duplex sonographic abnormalities in patients with renal artery stenosis. Ultrasound Quarterly 12:217–263, 1994.

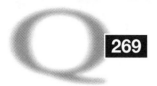

269

Which of the following terms can be
used to describe this waveform?

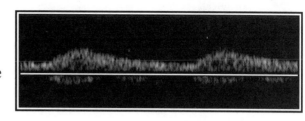

a. triphasic

b. biphasic

c. monophasic

d. multiphasic

A 269

C. Monophasic.

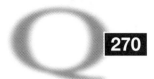

Both of these waveforms were obtained from segmental renal arteries in the renal hilum. Which waveform shows a normal resistance to flow?

a. top

b. bottom

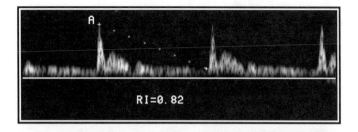

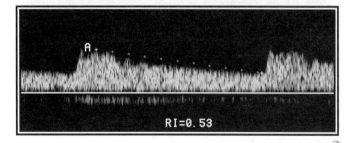

IV. Abdomen and Visceral / Testing and Treatment (4–13%)

A 270

A. Top.

The normal RI (resistive index) in the kidney is < 0.7. As the RI increases, the amount of diastolic flow will decrease. Normal waveforms obtained from the main renal artery or from arteries within the kidney are of low resistance with forward flow throughout the cardiac cycle. Increased resistance may be seen in cases of renal disease, renal vein thrombosis, and hematoma or other mass pressing upon the kidney.

▶ Stavros T, Harshfield D: Renal Doppler, renal artery stenosis, and renovascular hypertension: direct and indirect duplex sonographic abnormalities in patients with renal artery stenosis. Ultrasound Quarterly 12:217–263, 1994.

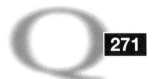

271

The pathology responsible for this abnormal waveform is most likely:

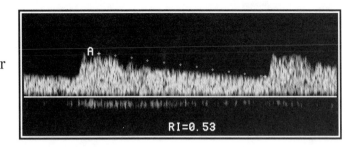

RI=0.53

a. renal artery stenosis

b. renal artery fibromuscular dysplasia

c. parenchymal renal disease

d. renal artery arteriovenous fistula

A 271

C. Parenchymal renal disease.

Q 272

Increased diastolic flow is seen in the superior mesenteric artery with which of the following?

a. postprandial state

b. stenosis

c. replaced hepatic artery

d. all of the above

A 272

D. All of the above.

The SMA will show low-resistance flow in the postprandial state, when stenosis is present or when variant anatomy such as a replaced hepatic artery arises from the proximal SMA.

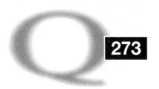

273

All of the arteries below demonstrate low-resistance waveforms in the fasting state **EXCEPT:**

a. inferior mesenteric artery

b. hepatic artery

c. splenic artery

d. renal artery

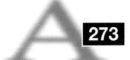

A. Inferior mesenteric artery.

Arteries that feed parenchymal organs—including the celiac, hepatic, splenic, and renal arteries in the abdomen—demonstrate low-resistance waveforms with forward flow present throughout the entire cardiac cycle. The superior and inferior mesenteric arteries show little diastolic flow in the fasting state. Following a meal, the diastolic flow in the superior mesenteric artery flow increases as much as 3 times its fasting level.

▶ Baxter BT, Pearce WH: Diagnosis and surgical management of chronic mesenteric ischemia. In Strandness DE, van Breda A (eds): *Vascular Diseases: Surgical and Interventional Therapy.* New York, Churchill Livingstone, 1994, pp 795–802.

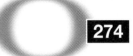

Q 274

What is the most common anatomic location of renal allografts?

a. left iliac fossa

b. right iliac fossa

c. mid pelvis

d. Morrison's pouch

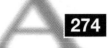
274

B. Right iliac fossa.

Most renal allografts (transplants) are located in the right lower quadrant.

▶ Rumwell C, McPharlin M: *Vascular Technology: An Illustrated Review,* 2nd edition. Pasadena, Davies Publishing, 2000, p 107.

275

The median arcuate ligament syndrome most commonly involves which vessel?

a. superior mesenteric artery
b. inferior mesenteric artery
c. portal vein
d. celiac trunk

A 275

D. Celiac trunk.

The median arcuate ligament syndrome usually involves only the celiac trunk, although rarely it may also compress the superior mesenteric artery as well.

▶ Matsumoto AH, Muehle C, Casada D, et al: Compression of the superior mesenteric artery by the median arcuate ligament: a cause for mesenteric ischemia. Vascular Surgery 28:489–493, 1994.

Q 276

Which of the following is a limitation of direct Doppler interrogation of the renal arteries?

a. stenosis in accessory renal arteries may not be detected

b. Doppler angles less than 60° may be difficult to obtain at the renal artery origins

c. patient body habitus can limit access to the renal arteries

d. all of the above

A 276

D. All of the above.

There are two methods for detecting renal artery stenosis with Doppler ultrasound, a direct and indirect method. The direct method involves Doppler interrogation throughout the length of each renal artery. Limitations of the technique include the high incidence of multiple renal arteries (as many as 25% of patients), difficulty obtaining adequate Doppler angles to the renal artery origins, and difficulty completely visualizing the renal arteries due to bowel gas or patient body habitus. When multiple renal arteries are present, they are frequently difficult to visualize ultrasonographically. The indirect technique involves Doppler interrogation of the segmental or interlobar arteries within the kidney. This indirect evaluation overcomes the limitations of poor patient body habitus and inadequate Doppler angles. The presence of multiple renal arteries is not a problem with this technique since Doppler samplings are taken from the upper, mid, and lower poles of the kidney. Limitations of the indirect technique include the inability to distinguish between stenosis and total occlusion and the inability to detect stenoses less than 60% diameter reduction.

► Stavros T, Harshfield D: Renal Doppler, renal artery stenosis, and renovascular hypertension: direct and indirect duplex sonographic abnormalities in patients with renal artery stenosis. Ultrasound Quarterly 12:217–263, 1994.

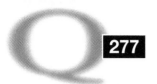

277

A 53-year-old male presents to the vascular lab with a 6-month history of severe hypertension and abdominal bruit. Which vessel is most likely the source of the patient's symptoms?

a. superior mesenteric artery

b. celiac trunk

c. renal artery

d. hepatic artery

A 277

C. Renal artery.

Q **278**

Which vessel would be imaged in a patient referred to rule out Budd-Chiari syndrome?

a. common femoral vein

b. innominate vein

c. internal jugular vein

d. hepatic vein

A 278

D. Hepatic vein.

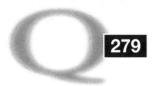

279

Which waveform (top or bottom) represents abnormal portal vein flow?

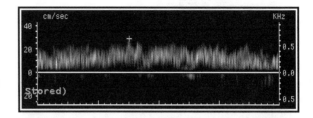

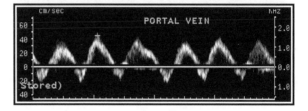

a. top

b. bottom

A 279

B. Bottom.

The normal waveform obtained from the portal vein is a mildly undulating signal. Prominent pulsatility or bidirectional flow as seen in bottom waveform is an abnormal finding and can be indicative of right heart failure, tricuspid regurgitation, portal vein–hepatic artery fistula, portal hypertension, and other abnormalities.

▶ Rosenthal SJ, Harrison LA, Baxter KG, et al: Doppler US of helical flow in the portal vein. Radiographics 15:1103–1111,1995.

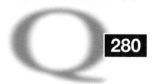

280

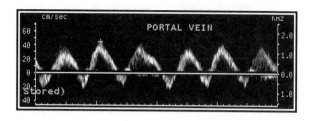

This abnormal portal venous
waveform may be indicative of:

a. tricuspid regurgitation

b. hepatic metastases

c. hepatic artery thrombosis

d. hepatic infarction

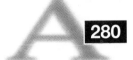

A. Tricuspid regurgitation.

A pulsatile portal vein waveform can result from right heart failure, tricuspid regurgitation, portal vein–hepatic artery fistula, portal hypertension, and other abnormalities.

▶ Rosenthal SJ, Harrison LA, Baxter KG, et al: Doppler US of helical flow in the portal vein. Radiographics 15:1103–1111,1995.

Q 281

Which of the following is a normal finding in a patient following a transjugular intra-hepatic portosystemic shunt (TIPS) procedure?

a. hepatofugal flow in the main portal vein
b. hepatofugal flow in intrahepatic portal radicles
c. hepatofugal flow in the splenic vein
d. all of the above

A 281

B. Hepatofugal flow in intrahepatic portal radicles.

Hepatofugal flow in the intrahepatic portal vein branches is a common finding following successful TIPS because flow follows the path of least resistance. Scarring in the liver due to cirrhosis results in high resistance to flow through intrahepatic portal branches. The TIPS stent produces a path of low resistance so flow in the portal branches reverses and courses toward the stent.

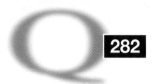

282

During the Valsalva maneuver, what happens to pressure in the abdomen and thorax?

a. intrathoracic pressure increases, abdominal pressure increases
b. intrathoracic pressure decreases, abdominal pressure decreases
c. intrathoracic pressure increases, abdominal pressure decreases
d. intrathoracic pressure decreases, abdominal pressure increases

IV. Abdomen and Visceral / Testing and Treatment (4–13%)

A 282

A. Intrathoracic pressure increases, abdominal pressure increases.

▶ Rumwell C, McPharlin M: *Vascular Technology: An Illustrated Review,* 2nd edition. Pasadena, Davies Publishing, 2000, p 181.

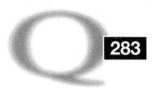

283

During inspiration, what happens to pressure in the abdomen and thorax?

a. Intrathoracic pressure increases, abdominal pressure increases.

b. Intrathoracic pressure decreases, abdominal pressure decreases.

c. Intrathoracic pressure increases, abdominal pressure decreases.

d. Intrathoracic pressure decreases, abdominal pressure increases.

A 283

D. Intrathoracic pressure decreases, abdominal pressure increases.

▶ Rumwell C, McPharlin M: *Vascular Technology: An Illustrated Review,* 2nd edition. Pasadena, Davies Publishing, 2000, p 181.

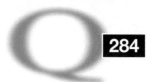

284

A 57-year-old female with a history of long-term alcohol abuse is referred for a portal venous duplex exam. The main portal vein cannot be identified at the porta hepatis, but instead multiple channels with hepatopetal flow are seen. This is consistent with:

a. caput medusae

b. cavernous transformation

c. paraumbilical flow

d. portal-hepatic fistula

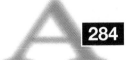

B. Cavernous transformation.

In cases of portal vein thrombosis, recanalization may occur, producing an appearance of multiple channels of hepatopetal flow within the porta hepatis instead of one main portal vein. This is termed *cavernous transformation of the portal vein.*

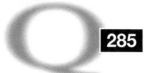

285

Which is **NOT** a sonographic finding associated with portal hypertension?

a. splenomegaly

b. gallbladder wall varices

c. ascites

d. lymphadenopathy

A 285

D. Lymphadenopathy.

Lymphadenopathy is not associated with portal hypertension. Splenomegaly is almost always present in cases of portal hypertension. Gallbladder wall varices are a less common feature but have a clear association. Ascites is frequently present and should increase suspicion for the presence of portal vein thrombosis.

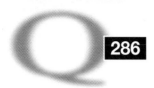

286

A patient in a hypercoagulable state is seen to have thrombosis of the right renal vein by duplex sonography. What other findings may be seen in association with this?

a. thrombus within the inferior vena cava

b. decreased diastolic flow in the right renal artery

c. poor visualization of interlobular flow by color Doppler

d. all of the above

A **286**

D. All of the above.

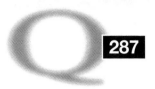

287

The normal waveform of the renal vein can be described as:

a. highly pulsatile
b. flat and continuous
c. phasic with respiration
d. triphasic

IV. Abdomen and Visceral / Testing and Treatment (4–13%)

287

C. Phasic with respiration.

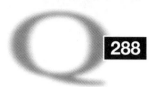

288

A spontaneous splenorenal shunt is an abnormal connection between the splenic and left renal vein and is associated with:

a. renovascular hypertension

b. portal hypertension

c. renal failure

d. renal cell carcinoma

A 288

B. Portal hypertension.

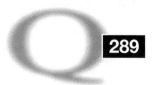

289

For saphenous vein mapping, which transducer would be the best choice?

a. 5 MHz linear array

b. 3 MHz curved array

c. 7–10 MHz linear array

d. 4–6 MHz curved array

A 289

C. 7–10 MHz linear array.

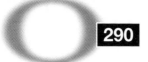

290

You are mapping the saphenous vein in a patient scheduled for coronary artery bypass surgery. You have discovered that the saphenous veins are inadequate for harvesting. Which of the following veins would be best to evaluate as an alternate graft?

a. cephalic vein

b. deep femoral vein

c. popliteal vein

d. axillary vein

DAVIES
Registry Reviews & Study Aids

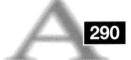

A. Cephalic vein.

The lesser saphenous, cephalic, and/or basilic veins may be mapped as possible conduits for bypass surgery when the saphenous vein is too small, diseased, or absent. Deep veins such as the deep femoral, popliteal, or axillary vein are not used.

Q 291

You have been asked to perform a vein mapping of the saphenous vein. Which of the following techniques would be most helpful?

a. Decrease the room temperature so the small saphenous vein will become dilated.

b. Place the patient in an upright position to improve visualization of the saphenous vein.

c. Place the patient in a prone position to improve access to the saphenous vein.

d. Use a high-frequency probe and light probe pressure to track the saphenous vein.

A 291

D. Use a high-frequency probe and light probe pressure to track the saphenous vein.

The highest-frequency linear array probe available should be used to track the saphenous vein because it is very superficial. Very light probe pressure should be used since it is easy to compress the vein by resting the probe on the skin. When the vein cannot be visualized, decreasing probe pressure will often help to demonstrate the vein. If the room temperature is too cold, the veins will be small and hard to see. The patient should be placed in a supine position with the leg externally rotated and the knee slightly bent.

▶ Talbot SR: Venous imaging technique. In Talbot SR, Oliver MA: *Techniques of Venous Imaging.* Pasadena, Davies Publishing, 1992, pp 59–118.

Q 292

A patient presents with a pseudoaneurysm following arterial puncture. For ultrasound-guided compression of the pseudoaneurysm, how long would each compression last before checking for cessation of flow into the pseudoaneurysm?

a. 1 minute

b. 10 minutes

c. 30 minutes

d. 45 minutes

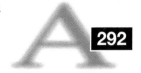

292

B. 10 minutes.

Repair of pseudoaneurysm by ultrasound-guided compression is accomplished by applying pressure with the ultrasound transducer over the neck of the pseudoaneurysm. Pressure is increased until a cessation of flow is apparent within the pseudoaneurysm while maintaining flow within the native artery. Multiple compressions lasting approximately 10 minutes each are usually necessary to obliterate the flow within the pseudoaneurysm and its communicating channel.

▶ Rumwell C, McPharlin M: *Vascular Technology: An Illustrated Review,* 2nd edition. Pasadena, Davies Publishing, 2000, pp 119–120.
▶ Hertz SM, Brener BJ: Ultrasound-guided pseudoaneurysm compression: efficacy after coronary stenting and angioplasty. J Vasc Surg 26:913–918, 1997.

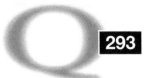

293

Arteriovenous fistula is a complication that most commonly occurs with:

a. reversed vein bypass grafts

b. in situ grafts

c. atherectomy

d. angioplasty

A 293

B. In situ grafts.

Arteriovenous fistula is not a complication of reversed vein bypass grafts, atherectomy, or angioplasty. It is a complication of in situ bypass grafts. Arteriovenous fistulas occur when one of the venous branches of the saphenous vein is not ligated, resulting in communication between the graft and an adjacent vein.

▶ Polak JF: Arterial sonography: efficacy for the diagnosis of arterial disease of the lower extremity. AJR 161:235–243, 1993.

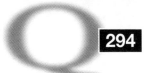

Q 294

What type of aneurysm is related to arterial trauma whereby blood escapes through a defect in the vessel wall and extravasates into the surrounding tissue?

a. fusiform aneurysm

b. saccular aneurysm

c. dissecting aneurysm

d. pseudoaneurysm

A **294**

D. Pseudoaneurysm.

▶ Rumwell C, McPharlin M: *Vascular Technology: An Illustrated Review,* 2nd edition. Pasadena, Davies Publishing, 2000, pp 37–38.

Q 295

A patient presents with swelling around the puncture site of arteriography. Duplex sonography reveals a high-velocity tract from the artery leading to a large hematoma. This is termed a(n):

a. dissection

b. arteriovenous fistula

c. pseudoaneurysm

d. subintimal hematoma

DAVIES
Registry Reviews & Study Aids

A **295**

C. Pseudoaneurysm.

296

Which of the following describes a typical venous Doppler waveform obtained proximal to an arteriovenous fistula?

a. continuous low velocity
b. prominent respiratory phasicity
c. increased velocity and pulsatility
d. unchanged from normal

A 296

C. Increased velocity and pulsatility.

Q 297

Which of the following describes a typical arterial Doppler waveform obtained proximal to an arteriovenous fistula?

a. high resistance with no diastolic flow

b. triphasic

c. low resistance with increased flow

d. bidirectional with increase velocities during systole and reverse flow in diastole

A 297

C. Low resistance with increased flow.

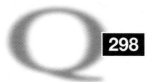
298

Which statement regarding arteriovenous fistula is **NOT** true?

a. Blood pressure in the distal artery is always increased.
b. A fistula located close to the heart increases the potential for cardiac failure.
c. Arterial flow proximal to the fistula is markedly increased.
d. A thrill may be felt over the fistula site.

A 298

A. This statement—"blood pressure in the distal artery is always increased"—is NOT true.

The blood pressure in the distal artery is always decreased in the presence of an arteriovenous fistula.

▶ Rumwell C, McPharlin M: *Vascular Technology: An Illustrated Review,* 2nd edition. Pasadena, Davies Publishing, 2000, p 113.

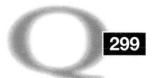

299

Which of the following describes the classic flow pattern in the neck of a traumatic pseudoaneurysm?

a. low resistance with high-velocity flow during systole
b. high resistance with absence of flow in diastole
c. trickle flow
d. high-velocity antegrade flow in systole with retrograde flow in diastole

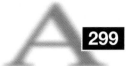

D. High-velocity antegrade flow in systole with retrograde flow in diastole.

The classic flow pattern in the neck of a pseudoaneurysm is bidirectional. Since blood tends to flow from high pressure to low pressure, it flows into the pseudoaneurysm in systole and back into the native artery during diastole.

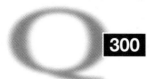

300

Your ultrasonographic findings in the lower extremity of a patient who has undergone cardiac catheterization include low-resistance, high-velocity flow in the common femoral artery and pulsatile flow in the common femoral vein. A prominent bruit is present. These findings are most closely associated with:

a. traumatic arteriovenous fistula

b. pseudoaneurysm

c. arterial dissection

d. arterial and venous compression due to hematoma

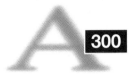

A. Traumatic arteriovenous fistula.

Arteriovenous fistula is an abnormal direct connection between an artery and vein. Fistulas may occur as complications of arterial puncture. When a fistula is present, arterial flow will be preferentially shunted into the low-pressure venous system. This will cause pulsatility in the downstream component of the affected vein. Since much of the arterial flow is coursing directly into the low resistance venous system, increased diastolic flow and high velocities will be seen in the artery proximal to the fistula.

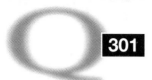

301

A Brescia-Cimino fistula is a type of:

a. dialysis access anastomosis

b. traumatic fistula

c. surgical correction for thoracic outlet syndrome

d. congenital fistula

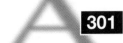

301

A. Dialysis access anastomosis.

This arteriovenous fistula between the radial artery and the cephalic vein is the preferred permanent vascular access for hemodialysis due to its fewer complications and greater longevity compared to other types of accesses.

▶ Finlay DI, Longley DG, Foshager MC, et al: Duplex and color Doppler sonography of hemodialysis arteriovenous fistulas and grafts. Radiographics 13:983–999,1993.

Q 302

This waveform is a typical example of the Doppler signal obtained from a(n):

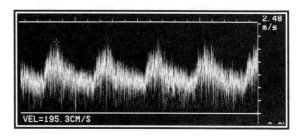

a. pseudoaneurysm neck

b. dialysis access graft

c. lower extremity arterial bypass graft

d. aneurysmal artery

A 302

B. Dialysis access graft.

Because a dialysis graft forms a direct fistula between an artery and a vein, the arterial signal will have high diastolic velocities reflecting the low resistance in the draining vein. Typical systolic velocities range between 100 and 400 cm/sec.

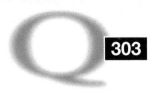

303

Which is a complication of dialysis access grafts?

a. arterial steal

b. aneurysm

c. venous stenosis

d. all of the above

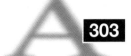

D. All of the above.

Complications of dialysis access grafts include arterial and venous stenoses, graft thrombosis, infection, aneurysm, and pseudoaneurysm formation, arterial steal, and hematoma.

▶ Finlay DI, Longley DG, Foshager MC, et al: Duplex and color Doppler sonography of hemodialysis arteriovenous fistulas and grafts. Radiographics 13:983–999,1993.

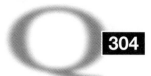

304

The location of the arterial anastomosis of the native common hepatic artery to the donor hepatic artery in liver transplants is:

a. in the posterior aspect of the right lobe of the liver

b. medial segment of the left lobe of the liver

c. several centimeters proximal to the hepatic hilum

d. at the porta hepatis where the hepatic artery enters the liver

A 304

C. Several centimeters proximal to the hepatic hilum.

▶ Foley WD: *Color Doppler Flow Imaging.* Boston, Andover Medical Publishers, 1991.

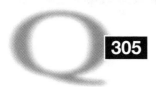

305

Which Doppler frequency would most likely be used to evaluate the penile artery?

a. 8 MHz

b. 20 MHz

c. 4 MHz

d. 2 MHz

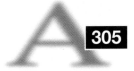

305

A. 8 MHz.

▶ Rumwell C, McPharlin M: *Vascular Technology: An Illustrated Review,* 2nd edition. Pasadena, Davies Publishing, 2000, p 68.

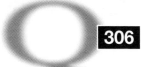

Which of the following represents a normal penile/brachial index (PBI)?

a. 0.75 or greater
b. 0.65–0.74
c. less than 0.65
d. all are normal

V. Miscellaneous Conditions and Tests (5–15%)

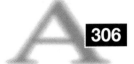
306

A. 0.75 or greater.

A normal PBI is 0.75 or greater. The calculation is based on the highest brachial pressure.

▶ Rumwell C, McPharlin M: *Vascular Technology: An Illustrated Review,* 2nd edition. Pasadena, Davies Publishing, 2000, p 67.

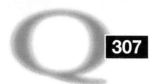

What is an advantage of using the radial artery over the saphenous vein for coronary artery bypass grafts?

a. vessel caliber similar to that of coronary arteries

b. thicker vessel wall

c. longer patency rates

d. all of the above

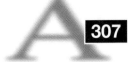

307

D. All of the above.

All of these are potential advantages of using the radial artery over the saphenous vein for coronary artery bypass grafts. An additional advantage is that many patients do not have adequate saphenous veins for harvesting due to prior thrombus, small size, or prior use.

▶ Winkler J, Lohr J, Bukhari RH, et al: Evaluation of the radial artery for use in coronary artery bypass grafting. J Vasc Technol 22:23–29, 1998.

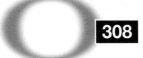

Q 308

The internal mammary artery is a branch of which of the following arteries?

a. innominate

b. subclavian

c. vertebral

d. axillary

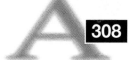

308

B.   Subclavian.

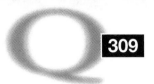

309

A common feature of temporal arteritis is:

a. dissection

b. aneurysm

c. intimal thickening

d. tortuosity

e. ectasia

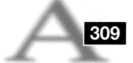

309

C. Intimal thickening.

Temporal arteritis causes marked thickening of the intima. It may be localized, focal, or widespread. Patients tend to present with severe headache. Other symptoms may include scalp tenderness, visual disturbance, joint pain, and painful chewing. Blindness can occur as a result of ischemic optic neuropathy in fewer than 20% of patients.

▶ Beers MH, Berkow R (eds): *The Merck Manual,* 17th ed. Whitehouse Station, NJ, Merck.

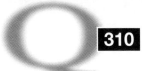

310

Which of the following describes the Adson maneuver used in diagnosis of thoracic outlet syndrome?

a. The patient hyperabducts the arm in conjunction with rapid opening and closing of the hand.

b. The patient's arm is at a 90° angle to the torso with the head turned toward the affected side and then away from the affected side during deep inspiration.

c. The patient assumes a military posture with the shoulders braced down.

d. The patient sits straight and crosses the arms in front during deep inspiration.

A 310

B. The patient's arm is at a 90° angle to the torso with the head turned toward the affected side and then away from the affected side during deep inspiration.

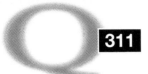

311

Symptoms associated with thoracic outlet syndrome include all of the following **EXCEPT:**

a. increased blood pressure on the affected side
b. numbness or tingling of the arm
c. aching of shoulder and forearm
d. increased discomfort with upward arm positions

A 311

A. Increased blood pressure on the affected side.

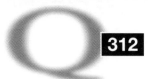

Q 312

Which of the following would **NOT** be associated with arterial trauma?

a. dissection

b. hematoma

c. pseudoaneurysm

d. fibromuscular dysplasia

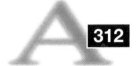 **312**

D. Fibromuscular dysplasia.

Fibromuscular dysplasia is a condition in which a series of small dilatations and narrowings occurs in an artery, creating an angiographic pattern referred to as a "string of pearls." It is more commonly seen in females and young individuals, but is not associated with arterial trauma. Dissection results from an intimal tear in an artery and may be caused by trauma or other factors such as fibromuscular dysplasia, hypertension, and Marfan's syndrome. A hematoma is simply a swelling caused by a mass of blood (usually clotted) resulting from a tear in a blood vessel. A pseudoaneurysm may also be a result of arterial trauma. It occurs when there is a tear in a vessel with blood leaking out into a space that is not confined by the vessel wall. An arterial track with bidirectional flow is seen leading from the artery to the pulsing hematoma.

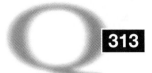

313

You are performing a Doppler exam on a 32-year-old female who was recently involved in a car accident. She received a blow to the left side of her body. She presents with an abdominal bruit, back pain, and hypertension. Which of the following conditions is most likely?

a. fibromuscular dysplasia involving the splenic and common hepatic arteries

b. Takaysu's arteritis involving the abdominal aorta

c. dissection involving the abdominal aorta and possibly the renal arteries

d. inflammatory aneurysm of the infrarenal abdominal aorta

A 313

C. Dissection involving the abdominal aorta and possibly the renal arteries.

Of the conditions listed, only arterial dissection is related to trauma. Dissection of the abdominal aorta can compromise flow to the renal arteries resulting in hypertension. Dissection may even extend into the renal arteries and compromise flow.

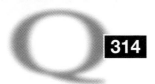

314

You are performing an ultrasound exam on a patient with a gunshot wound involving the posterior tibial artery. What artifact is associated with metallic objects such as bullets?

a. Enhancement
b. Multipath
c. Comet tail
d. Mirror image

A 314

C. Comet tail.

Comet tail artifacts are associated with metallic objects such as bullets or surgical clips. The appearance of a comet tail artifact is a series of bands underneath the metallic object. The artifact is caused by multiple reverberations of the sound wave within the tiny metallic structure.

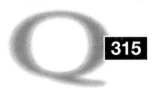

315

The ability of a noninvasive test to detect disease when it is present is termed:

a. sensitivity

b. specificity

c. accuracy

d. negative predictive value

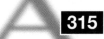

315

A. Sensitivity.

Calculation: True positives ÷ True positives + False negatives.

▶ Rumwell C, McPharlin M: *Vascular Technology: An Illustrated Review,* 2nd edition. Pasadena, Davies Publishing, 2000, pp 215–221.

Q 316

The ability of a noninvasive test to identify that no disease is present when there is no disease is termed:

a. sensitivity
b. specificity
c. accuracy
d. positive predictive value

A **316**

B. Specificity.

Calculation: True negatives $\div$ True negatives + False positives.

▶ Rumwell C, McPharlin M: *Vascular Technology: An Illustrated Review,* 2nd edition. Pasadena, Davies Publishing, 2000, pp 215–221.

Q 317

Which of the following is calculated by dividing the total number of correct tests by the total number of all tests?

a. sensitivity
b. specificity
c. accuracy
d. positive predictive value

317

C. Accuracy.

Accuracy is the percentage of correct diagnoses made by the noninvasive test.

▶ Rumwell C, McPharlin M: *Vascular Technology: An Illustrated Review,* 2nd edition. Pasadena, Davies Publishing, 2000, pp 215–221.

Q 318

The number of true positives divided by the number of true positives + false positives describes which of the following?

a. sensitivity

b. specificity

c. accuracy

d. positive predictive value

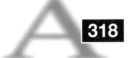

318

D. Positive predictive value.

The positive predictive value describes the percentage of individuals with a positive noninvasive test result who actually have the disease.

▶   Rumwell C, McPharlin M: *Vascular Technology: An Illustrated Review,* 2nd edition. Pasadena, Davies Publishing, 2000, pp 215–221.

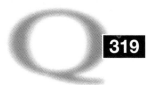

319

The proportion of test results that correctly predict normality is termed:

a. sensitivity
b. specificity
c. accuracy
d. negative predictive value

A 319

D. Negative predictive value.

Calculation: True negatives ÷ True negatives + False negatives.

▶ Rumwell C, McPharlin M: *Vascular Technology: An Illustrated Review,* 2nd edition. Pasadena, Davies Publishing, 2000, pp 215–221.

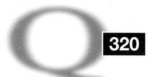

320

If the noninvasive test results were positive, but the gold standard showed normal results, the noninvasive test results are referred to as:

a. false positive
b. false negative
c. true positive
d. true negative

320

A. False positive.

A false-positive test is one in which the noninvasive test results were positive but the gold standard test results were negative (i.e., normal).

▶ Rumwell C, McPharlin M: *Vascular Technology: An Illustrated Review,* 2nd edition. Pasadena, Davies Publishing, 2000, pp 215–221.

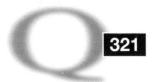

321

The best way to prepare a transducer for intraoperative use is:

a. autoclave

b. immerse for 72 hours in Cidex solution

c. soap and water

d. place transducer and acoustic gel within a sterile sleeve or bag

A 321

D. Place transducer and acoustic gel within a sterile sleeve or bag,

Autoclaving a transducer will destroy its piezoelecteric properties.

Q 322

According to Poiseuille's law, what would occur to the pressure gradient across an arterial segment in which the radius has been reduced by ½?

a. no effect

b. increase

c. decrease

d. not enough information to determine

A 322

B. Increase.

Q 323

The tendency of objects to maintain their status quo is called:

a. kinetic energy
b. potential energy
c. inertia
d. hydrostatic pressure

A 323

C. Inertia.

324

Where would a dampened Doppler signal be obtained?

a. A

b. B

c. C

d. none of the above

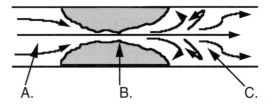

A.   B.   C.

648

A. A

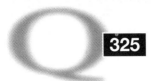

325

Where would a Doppler signal be obtained that showed spectral broadening?

a. A
b. B
c. C
d. none of the above

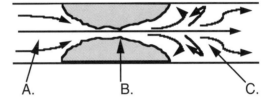

A.   B.   C.

650

A **325**

C. C

Q 326

Where would the lowest pressure be found?

a. A
b. B
c. C
d. none of the above

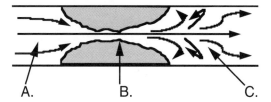

A.   B.   C.

A 326

B. B

▶ Kremkau FW: *Doppler Ultrasound.* Philadelphia, Saunders, 1990.

327

Where would the Reynolds number be greatest?

a. A

b. B

c. C

d. none of the above

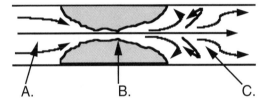

A.   B.   C.

VII. Physiology and Fluid Dynamics / Arterial Hemodynamics (7-11%)

327

C. C

Q 328

Where would the Doppler signal show the highest bandwidth?

a. A

b. B

c. C

d. none of the above

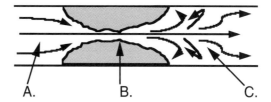

328

C. C

Q 329

Where would laminar flow be found?

a. A

b. B

c. C

d. none of the above

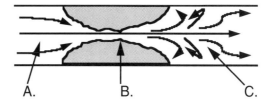

A 329

D. None of the above.

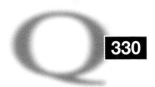

330

What term best describes the pulse profile in this illustration?

a. blunt

b. parabolic

c. flat

d. laminar

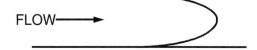

FLOW

660

A 330

B. Parabolic.

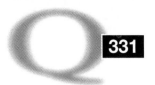

331

The resistance to flow offered by the fluid in motion is termed:

a. viscosity

b. pressure gradient

c. kinetic energy

d. inertia

A 331

A. Viscosity.

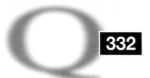

332

The Bernoulli effect describes:

a. decreased resistance distal to a stenosis

b. decreased pressure in regions of high flow speed

c. decreased velocities in regions of flow turbulence

d. decreased flow volume in critical stenosis

A 332

B.   Decreased pressure in regions of high flow speed.

Q 333

Why do collateral vessels tend to have higher resistance than normal flow channels?

a. small lumen diameter

b. greater length

c. higher viscosity

d. a and b

666

D. A and B.

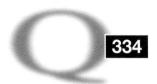

334

What is the effect of massage or pressure on the carotid sinus?

a. increase blood pressure
b. tachycardia
c. increase stroke volume
d. reflex bradycardia

A **334**

D. Reflex bradycardia.

▶ Belanger AC: *Vascular Anatomy and Physiology.* Pasadena, Davies Publishing, 1999, p 75.

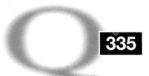

335

Peripheral resistance is controlled by:

a. muscle contraction
b. vasoconstriction and vasodilatation of the arterioles
c. stroke volume
d. heart rate

335

B. Vasoconstriction and vasodilatation of the arterioles.

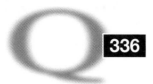

336

The energy of something in motion is termed:

a. kinetic energy
b. potential energy
c. fluid energy
d. viscous energy

A **336**

A. Kinetic energy.

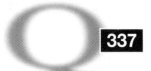

337

What changes would be seen in a Doppler waveform of the femoral artery that is taken after exercise?

a. no changes

b. increased flow throughout diastole

c. increased reverse component in early diastole

d. delayed systolic rise time

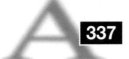

337

B. Increased flow throughout diastole.

During exercise, the muscles have greater demand for oxygenated blood. The arterioles dilate and resistance to flow decreases. As flow resistance diminishes, the volume of diastolic flow increases.

▶ Belanger AC: *Vascular Anatomy and Physiology.* Pasadena, Davies Publishing, 1999, pp 163–165.

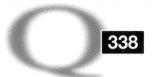

338

The Reynolds number denotes the:

a. effect of pressure on volume flow

b. effect of arteriolar vasodilation or vasoconstriction on flow velocity

c. point at which resistance to flow is increased in a stenosis

d. point at which flow becomes turbulent

A 338

D. Point at which flow becomes turbulent.

Q 339

What factor has the greatest influence on flow resistance?

a. viscosity

b. vessel radius

c. vessel length

d. pressure gradient

339

B. Vessel radius.

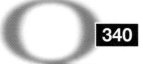

340

The term *laminar flow* describes the:

a. layered manner in which blood flow courses within an arterial lumen

b. turbulent flow distal to a stenosis

c. accelerated flow within a narrowed arterial segment

d. disturbed flow at arterial bifurcations

A **340**

A. Layered manner in which blood flow courses within an arterial lumen.

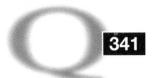

341

Which of the following accurately describes the exit effects of flow through a stenosis?

a. The flow profile elongates and eventually reestablishes as parabolic.

b. Boundary layer separation occurs.

c. Flow near the vessel edges becomes stagnant or retrograde.

d. all of the above

A **341**

D. All of the above.

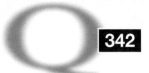

342

A plug flow profile would most likely be seen in which vessels?

a. external carotid artery

b. vertebral artery

c. proper hepatic artery

d. abdominal aorta

A 342

D. Abdominal aorta.

A plug or blunted flow profile is seen in large arteries such as the abdominal aorta and common carotid artery. In these arteries the central portion of the fluid moves together and a velocity gradient occurs near the wall.

▶ Belanger AC: *Vascular Anatomy and Physiology.* Pasadena, Davies Publishing, 1999, pp 123–125.

Q 343

The term *phasicity,* in reference to the venous system, refers to:

a. the influence of the cardiac cycle on venous flow
b. the rate at which the valves open and close
c. the ebb and flow in the veins that occurs in response to respiration
d. the effect of intrinsic and extrinsic pressure on venous wall stiffness

A 343

C. The ebb and flow in the veins that occurs in response to respiration.

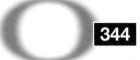

344

Which position would result in the greatest hydrostatic pressure?

a. Trendelenburg

b. supine

c. standing

d. Hydrostatic pressure does not vary with position.

A 344

C. Standing.

Hydrostatic pressure varies with position. It is the pressure exerted by fluid within a closed system, such as oil in a pipeline or blood in the circulatory system. Hydrostatic pressure is greatest in a standing position. In a supine position there is virtually no hydrostatic pressure.

▶ Belanger AC: *Vascular Anatomy and Physiology.* Pasadena, Davies Publishing, 1999, pp 131, 173–175.

Q 345

What is the effect of inspiration on venous flow in the lower extremities?

a. During inspiration the flow courses from the perforating veins into the superficial veins.

b. If the calf muscle is contracted, the flow will course toward the ankle during inspiration.

c. With competent valves, venous flow augments during inspiration and reverses during expiration.

d. In the supine position, venous flow in the lower extremities stops during inspiration and returns during expiration.

A 345

D. In the supine position, venous flow in the lower extremities stops during inspiration and returns during expiration.

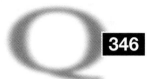

346

At any moment, how much of the body's blood volume is found in the veins?

a. 10–20%

b. 25–40%

c. 40–50%

d. 60–75%

A 346

D. 60–75%.

▶ Belanger AC: *Vascular Anatomy and Physiology*. Pasadena, Davies Publishing, 1999, p 167.

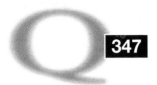

347

Which of the following would **NOT** be true regarding the lower extremity veins in an individual who has been standing for a long time?

a. The veins of the lower extremity would collapse under the increased pressure.

b. Hypotension could occur due to diminished cardiac output.

c. Hydrostatic pressure would be high in the lower extremity veins.

d. Pooling of blood would occur in the lower extremity veins.

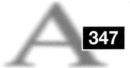

347

A. This statement—"the veins of the lower extremity would collapse under the increased pressure"—is NOT true.

In fact the veins of the lower extremity would become distended as a result of venous pooling and high pressure.

▶ Belanger AC: *Vascular Anatomy and Physiology.* Pasadena, Davies Publishing, 1999, pp 167–183.

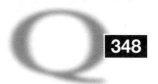

348

Which of the following would **NOT** be true regarding the calf muscle pump?

a. Contraction of the muscle propels blood toward the heart.

b. Hydrostatic pressure is increased in the veins at the ankle with contraction of the muscle pump.

c. Muscular contraction increases venous return and therefore cardiac output.

d. Competent valves stop blood from flowing retrograde during muscle contraction.

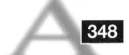

348

B. Hydrostatic pressure is increased in the veins at the ankle with contraction of the muscle pump.

With contraction of the calf muscle pump, the hydrostatic fluid column is interrupted and pressure is decreased in the veins at the ankle.

▶ Belanger AC: *Vascular Anatomy and Physiology.* Pasadena, Davies Publishing, 1999, pp 167–183.

349

Which statement is **NOT** true regarding intrathoracic pressure?

a. Intrathoracic pressure is increased with inspiration.

b. Venous return from the upper extremities is reduced when intrathoracic pressure is high.

c. Intrathoracic pressure is increased with the Valsalva maneuver.

d. Intrathoracic pressure has a major effect on venous return.

A 349

A. This statement—"intrathoracic pressure increases with inspiration"—is NOT true.

With inspiration, intrathoracic pressure decreases and intraabdominal pressure increases. This increases venous return from the upper extremity and stops venous flow in the lower extremity. The Valsalva maneuver increases both intrathoracic and intraabdominal pressure, which decreases venous return to the heart.

▶ Rumwell C, McPharlin M: *Vascular Technology: An Illustrated Review,* 2nd edition. Pasadena, Davies Publishing, 2000, p 181.

Q 350

The main power source for blood propulsion in the venous system is:

a. semilunar valves

b. right atrium

c. calf muscle

d. respiration

A 350

C. Calf muscle.

Q 351

A condition in which the body tissue contains excessive fluid is termed:

a. edema

b. pigmentation

c. cellulitis

d. lymphangitis

351

A. Edema.

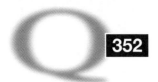

Q 352

Which of the following does **NOT** accurately describe events during calf muscle contraction and relaxation?

a. A potential "space" is created with very low pressure during relaxation.

b. Blood flows from the deep system into the superficial system via the perforators during relaxation.

c. Blood is forced cephalad during contraction.

d. Soleal sinuses empty during contraction.

DAVIES
Registry Reviews & Study Aids

A **352**

B. This statement—"blood flows from the deep system into the superficial system via the perforators during relaxation"—is NOT correct.

During relaxation, blood flows from the superficial system into the deep system.

▶ Rumwell C, McPharlin M: *Vascular Technology: An Illustrated Review,* 2nd edition. Pasadena, Davies Publishing, 2000, p 180.

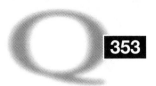

353

The veins lose their elliptical shape and become more circular with which of the following?

a. increased transmural pressure

b. increased interstitial pressure

c. decreased intraluminal pressure

d. decreased hydrostatic pressure

353

A. Increased transmural pressure.

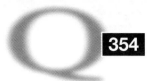

354

Which pressure is greatly influenced by gravity?

a. transmural pressure

b. interstitial pressure

c. intraluminal pressure

d. hydrostatic pressure

354

D. Hydrostatic pressure.

Q 355

Intraabdominal pressure is decreased with:

a. inspiration

b. expiration

c. Valsalva maneuver

d. a and c

355

B. Expiration.

Q 356

The ability of veins to accommodate large shifts in volume with only limited changes in venous pressure is known as:

a. augmentation
b. compliance
c. phasicity
d. transluminal pressure

A 356

B.   Compliance.

▶ Rumwell C, McPharlin M: *Vascular Technology: An Illustrated Review,* 2nd edition. Pasadena, Davies Publishing, 2000, pp 177–181.

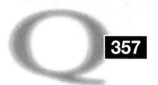

357

All of the changes below can be attributed to incompetent venous valves following venous thrombosis **EXCEPT**:

a. edema

b. venous hypertension

c. venous malformation

d. varicose superficial veins

A 357

C. Venous malformation.

With incompetent valves, the hydrostatic pressure column is uninterrupted from the right atrium to the lower legs. This pressure leads to venous distention and more incompetent veins in superficial veins and perforators. Secondary varicose veins develop. Edema, cellulitis, brown discoloration of the skin, and ulceration eventually may develop.

▶ Rumwell C, McPharlin M: *Vascular Technology: An Illustrated Review,* 2nd edition. Pasadena, Davies Publishing, 2000, pp 112–113, 179–180.

Q 358

All of the statements below are accurate regarding an arteriovenous fistula **EXCEPT:**

a. There is an increase in the volume of blood flow in the feeding artery.

b. Arterial resistance proximal to the fistula is decreased.

c. Venous pressure in draining veins is decreased.

d. High output cardiac failure is common in large arteriovenous fistulae.

358

C. Venous pressure in draining veins is decreased.

Q 359

What Doppler findings would **NOT** be evident in an acute traumatic arteriovenous fistula?

a. increased diastolic flow in the feeding artery

b. increased systolic velocity in the feeding artery

c. pulsatile flow in the draining vein

d. prominent collateral veins around the fistula

A 359

D. Prominent collateral veins around the fistula would NOT be evident in this situation.

In an acute setting, collateral vessels have not had time to develop. All other statements are true.

360

Which statement is **NOT** true regarding arteriovenous malformations?

a. They are present at birth.

b. They may be asymptomatic.

c. They can be defined as a direct connection between an artery and a vein.

d. They can occur anywhere in the body.

A 360

C. This statement—"they can be defined as a direct connection between an artery and a vein"—is NOT true.

An arteriovenous <u>fistula</u> is a direct communication between an artery and a vein. An arteriovenous <u>malformation</u> is present at birth and is an abnormal network in which arterial afferents flow directly into venous efferents without an intervening capillary bed.

Q 361

Complications associated with hemodialysis access grafts include all of the following **EXCEPT:**

a. distal limb ischemia

b. decreased distal venous pressure

c. pseudoaneurysm

d. congestive heart failure

A 361

B. Decreased distal venous pressure.

With hemodialysis access grafts, distal venous hypertension (not hypotension) may develop as a complication due to reversal of flow in the distal vein away from the fistula.

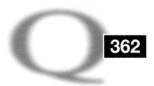

362

Which of the following does **NOT** occur as a result of trauma?

a. arteriovenous malformation
b. arteriovenous fistula
c. pseudoaneurysm
d. dissection

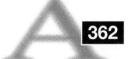

A. Arteriovenous malformation.

Arteriovenous fistulae, pseudoaneurysms, and dissections commonly occur as a result of trauma. An arteriovenous malformation may be exacerbated by trauma, but is present at birth.

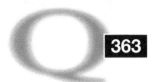

Q 363

In this image from a 48-year-old male, a large paraumbilical vein is seen exiting the liver. This is indicative of:

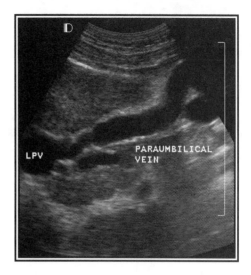

a. arteriovenous fistula between the hepatic and portal venous system

b. main portal vein thrombosis

c. portal hypertension

d. hepatofugal flow in the main portal vein

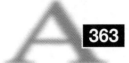

C. Portal hypertension.

Although not all patients with portal hypertension develop an enlarged paraumbilical vein, its presence is diagnostic of the disorder. The paraumbilical vein is a vestige of the umbilical circulation in the fetus. The paraumbilical vein(s) connects the portal venous system to the systemic venous system, forming a portosystemic shunt.

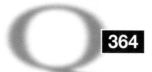

Q 364

The paraumbilical vein drains into a network of varices that can be seen on the abdomen radiating from the umbilicus. These varices are known as:

a. cavernous transformation

b. Caput Medusae

c. veins of Sappey

d. azygos veins

DAVIES
Registry Reviews & Study Aids

364

B.   Caput medusae.

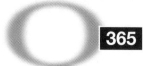

Q 365

This image is from a 64-year-old male with back pain. Which term best describes the aortic aneurysm?

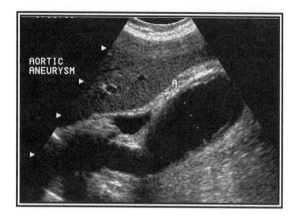

a. fusiform

b. saccular

c. mycotic

d. ectatic

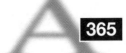

A. Fusiform.

A *fusiform* aneurysm is a circumferential enlargement of a segment of the artery and is the most common aneurysm shape. A *saccular* aneurysm is a focal out-pouching of an artery. A *mycotic* aneurysm is one that has become infected; the term "mycotic" does not describe a specific aneurysmal shape. An *ectatic* artery is one that is dilated but not aneurysmal by definition.

▶ Rumwell C, McPharlin M: *Vascular Technology: An Illustrated Review,* 2nd edition. Pasadena, Davies Publishing, 2000, pp 37–38.

Q 366

An aneurysm resulting from infection is termed:

a. fusiform

b. saccular

c. mycotic

d. ectatic

A 366

C. Mycotic.

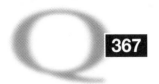

Q 367

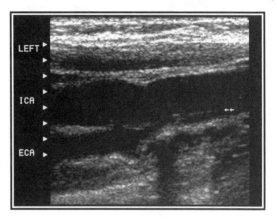

This image of the common carotid artery is from a 36-year-old female with Marfan's syndrome. The linear structure indicated by the arrows represents an intimal flap. Which of the following conditions is present?

a. pseudoaneurysm

b. arterial dissection

c. fibromuscular hyperplasia

d. arteriovenous fistula

DAVIES
Registry Reviews & Study Aids

A 367

B. Arterial dissection.

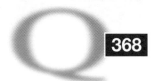

368

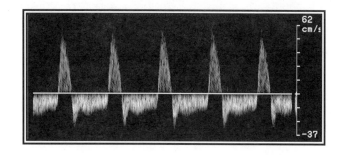

This image of the popliteal vein is from a 46-year-old female with leg swelling. Which of the following correctly describes the ultrasound findings?

a. Baker's cyst

b. acute thrombus in the popliteal vein

c. chronic thrombus in the popliteal vein

d. Rouleaux formation in the popliteal vein

A 368

B. Acute thrombus in the popliteal vein.

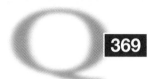

369

This waveform profile is characteristic of which of the following?

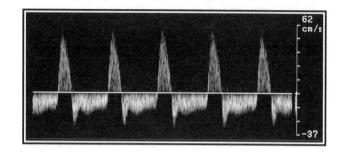

a. neck of pseudoaneurysm

b. arteriovenous communication

c. dampened signal obtained proximal to arterial occlusion

d. hyperemic flow

A **369**

A. Neck of pseudoaneurysm.

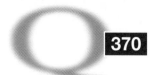

370

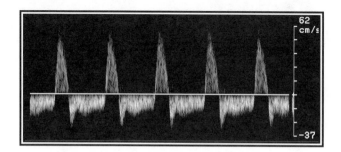

Which term can be used to describe this waveform?

a. monophasic
b. bidirectional
c. hepatofugal
d. tardus parvus

DAVIES
Registry Reviews & Study Aids

A 370

B. Bidirectional.

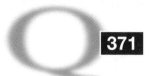

371

This waveform profile is characteristic of which of the following?

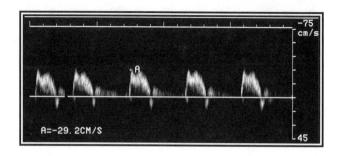

a. neck of pseudoaneurysm

b. arteriovenous communication

c. dampened signal obtained proximal to arterial occlusion

d. hyperemic flow

DAVIES
Registry Reviews & Study Aids

C. Dampened signal obtained proximal to arterial occlusion.

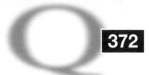

372

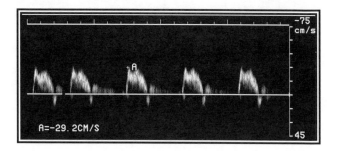

Which term can be used to
describe this waveform?

a. monophasic

b. biphasic

c. triphasic

d. tardus parvus

A 372

C. Triphasic.

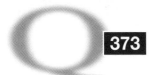

373

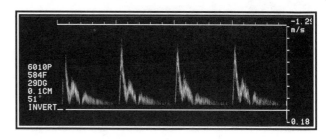

The end diastolic portion of this external carotid artery waveform is not demonstrated on this image because:

a. The pulse repetition frequency is set too low.

b. The wall filter is set too high.

c. The Doppler angle is too great.

d. The Doppler frequency is too high.

A 373

B. The wall filter is set too high.

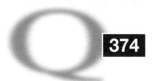

374

Which statement is **TRUE** regarding measurements obtained from this waveform?

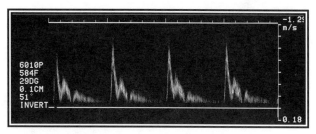

a. The resistive index would be erroneously high.

b. The pulsatility index would be erroneously low.

c. The acceleration time would be erroneously short.

d. The peak systolic velocity would be erroneously low.

A 374

A. The resistive index would be erroneously high.

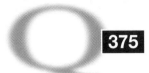

375

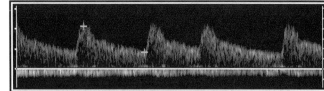

This waveform was obtained
at the porta hepatis in a patient
with portal hypertension. The
signals from both the portal vein
and hepatic artery are demonstrated.
Which of the following statements is correct?

a. The hepatic artery shows a high-resistance waveform pattern.

b. Hepatofugal flow is present in the portal vein.

c. Hepatofugal flow is present in the hepatic artery.

d. A fistula is present between the portal vein and hepatic artery.

A 375

B. Hepatofugal flow is present in the portal vein.

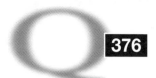

376

What clinical condition is associated with the findings seen in this waveform?

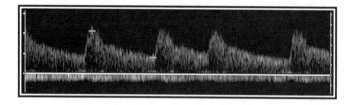

a. hepatic rejection

b. portal hypertension

c. right heart failure

d. hepatitis

A **376**

B. Portal hypertension.

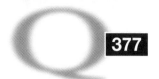

377

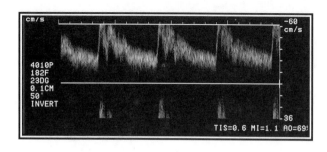

This waveform was obtained in the internal carotid artery. What technical problem is present?

a. Aliasing is present.

b. The baseline is set too low.

c. The wall filter is set too high.

d. The pulse repetition frequency is too high.

A. Aliasing is present.

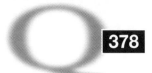

378

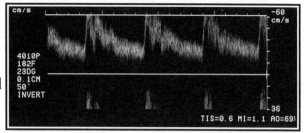

The technical problem demonstrated in this waveform could result in which of the following errors?

a. underestimation of end diastolic velocity

b. overestimation of acceleration time

c. overestimation of the resistive index

d. underestimation of peak systolic velocity

A 378

D. Underestimation of peak systolic velocity.

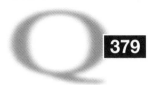

379

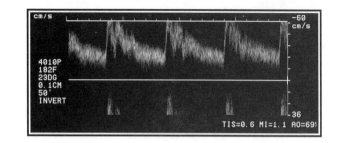

Which of the following would **NOT** correct the technical problem demonstrated in this waveform?

a. Lower the zero baseline.

b. Increase the pulse repetition frequency.

c. Decrease the wall filter.

d. Decrease the Doppler frequency.

758

A 379

C. Decrease the wall filter.

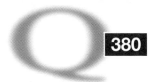

Q 380

This image is from a 22-year-old female with abnormal liver function tests and ascites. The thrombus in the inferior vena cava is most likely related to which of the following?

a. Budd-Chiari syndrome

b. Takayasu's arteritis

c. cavernous transformation

d. portal hypertension

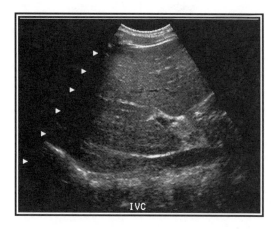

IVC

A 380

A. Budd-Chiari syndrome.

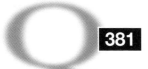

381

In the case described in question 380, which other abdominal vessel(s) should be evaluated for patency?

a. hepatic artery
b. portal vein
c. hepatic veins
d. b and c

762

A 381

D. B and C.

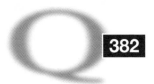

382

Name the vessels labeled A–C:

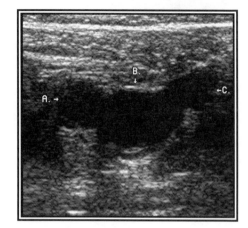

a. _____

b. _____

c. _____

A 382

A. Common femoral artery.

B. Common femoral vein.

C. Greater saphenous vein.

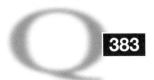

383

This image was taken:

a. in the neck

b. at the level of the knee

c. at the adductor canal

d. at the level of the inguinal ligament

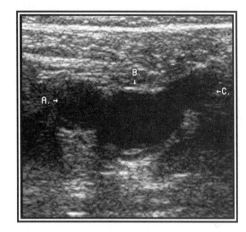

A 383

D. At the level of the inguinal ligament.

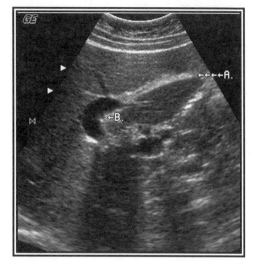

Q 384

Name the structures labeled A and B:

a. _____

b. _____

384

A. Left portal vein.
B. Ligamentum teres.

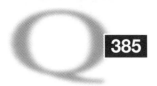

385

Which of the following conditions is ruled out by this image?

a. presence of a paraumbilical vein

b. cavernous transformation

c. hepatic vein thrombosis

d. splenic vein thrombosis

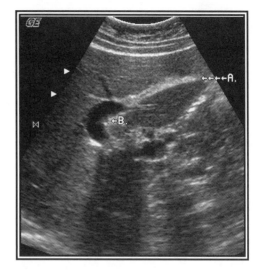

385

A. Presence of a paraumbilical vein.

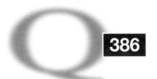

386

Name the vessels labeled A–C:

a. _____

b. _____

c. _____

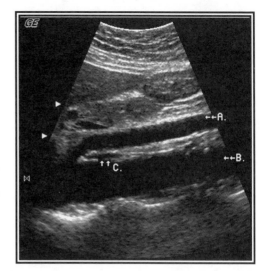

A 386

A. Superior mesenteric artery (SMA).

B. Abdominal aorta.

C. Left renal vein (LRV).

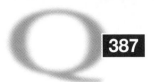

387

This image was obtained in which scan plane?

a. transverse

b. coronal

c. sagittal

d. oblique

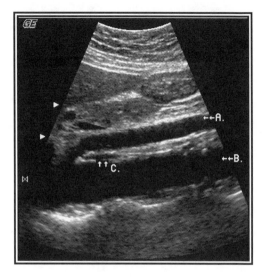

A 387

C. Sagittal.

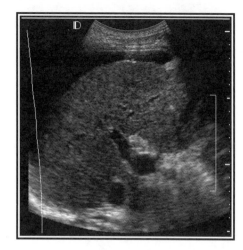

Q 388

This image is from a 48-year-old male with increasing abdominal girth and a history of alcohol abuse. Which condition is most likely?

a. portal hypertension

b. hepatic artery stenosis

c. Budd-Chiari syndrome

d. cavernous transformation of the portal vein

A 388

A. Portal hypertension.

Q 389

In this B-mode image, name the vessel seen in
cross section underneath the inferior vena cava.

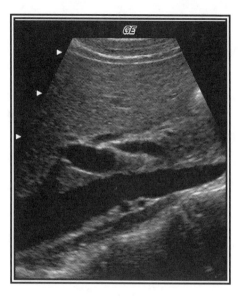

_____

DAVIES
Registry Reviews & Study Aids

A 389

Right renal artery.

The right renal artery passes underneath the inferior vena cava as it courses to the hilum of the kidney.

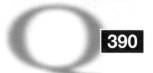

Q 390

In this B-mode image, what variant vascular anatomy is present?

_____

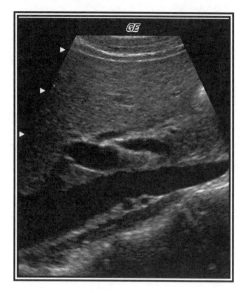

A 390

Multiple renal arteries.

There are two renal arteries in this image posterior to the inferior vena cava. Multiple renal arteries occur in up to 20% of individuals. When evaluating the renal arteries for stenosis in renovascular hypertension, each renal artery identified must be evaluated throughout its length. The presence of unidentified accessory or supernumerary renal arteries is a potential pitfall in the ultrasound evaluation for renal artery stenosis.

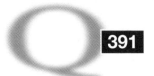

391

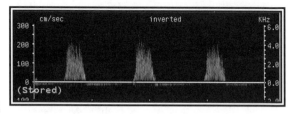

This Doppler waveform was obtained in a stenotic femoral artery. Was it most likely taken proximal or distal to the site of stenosis?

_____

A 391

Distal.

This waveform demonstrates poststenotic turbulence. This can be seen in the fill-in of the spectral window and the presence of a small amount of flow below the zero baseline.

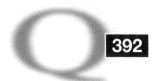

392

Which term can be used to describe
this waveform?

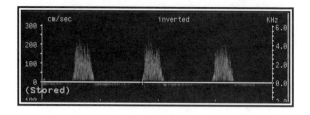

a. monophasic
b. spectral broadening
c. phasic
d. tardus parvus

A 392

B. Spectral broadening.

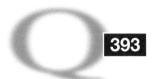

Q 393

What technical problem is present in this duplex sampling of the common carotid artery?

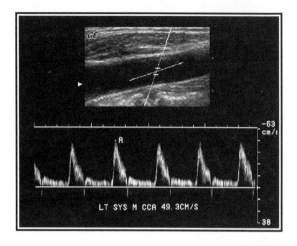

a. incorrect pulse repetition frequency

b. incorrect measurement of the Doppler angle

c. wall filter set incorrectly

d. Doppler gain too high

A 393

B. Incorrect measurement of the Doppler angle.

The Doppler angle should be aligned parallel to the vessel walls at the point of sampling.

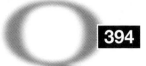

Q 394

What error could result from the technical problem shown in question 393?

a. underestimation of peak velocity

b. overestimation of peak velocity

c. erroneous display of spectral broadening

d. overestimation of systolic acceleration time

A 394

A. Underestimation of peak velocity.

Misalignment of the Doppler angle will result in inaccurate velocity calculations. If the measured angle is smaller than actual angle, the velocity will be underestimated. If the measured angle is larger than the actual angle, the velocity will be overestimated.

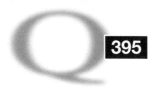

395

Name the vessels labeled A–D.

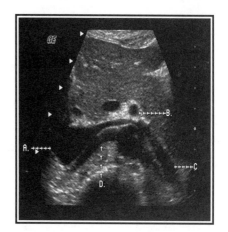

a. _____

b. _____

c. _____

d. _____

DAVIES
Registry Reviews & Study Aids

A 395

A. IVC.

B. SMA.

C. Left renal vein.

D. Right renal artery.

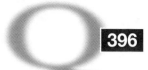

Q 396

This sagittal abdominal image shows a Greenfield filter positioned within what vessel?

a. portal vein

b. abdominal aorta

c. hepatic vein

d. inferior vena cava

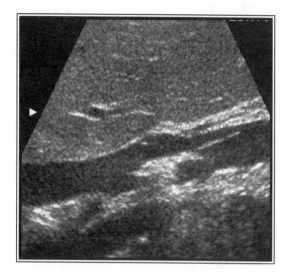

A **396**

D. Inferior vena cava.

397

Name the anatomy demonstrated adjacent to the aorta in this transverse image of an abdominal aortic aneurysm.

a. lymphadenopathy

b. retroperitoneal fibrosis

c. horseshoe kidneys

d. hematoma

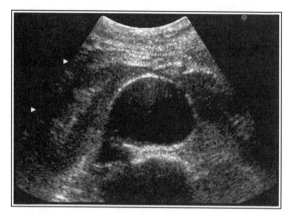

A 397

C. Horseshoe kidneys.

Horseshoe kidney is an anatomic variant in which both kidneys are connected at their lower (or, rarely, upper) poles across the midline. This can be a complicating factor in aortic surgery.

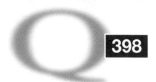

398

What term can be used to describe the atherosclerotic plaque in this sagittal image of the internal carotid artery?

a. homogeneous

b. smooth

c. heterogeneous

d. a and b

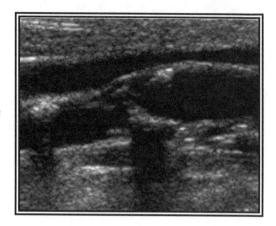

A 398

C. Heterogeneous.

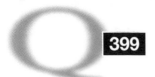

399

This waveform was most likely obtained from which abdominal vessel?

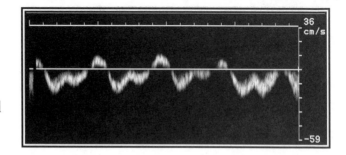

a. hepatic vein

b. portal vein

c. superior mesenteric vein

d. splenic vein

DAVIES
Registry Reviews & Study Aids

A **399**

A. Hepatic vein.

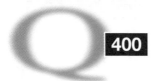

Q 400

This image was obtained just below the inguinal ligament in a 37-year-old female with leg swelling. Which of the following accurately describes the ultrasound findings?

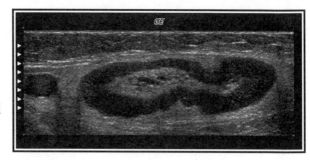

a. acute DVT of the common femoral vein

b. reactive lymph nodes

c. Baker's cyst

d. thigh sarcoma

DAVIES
Registry Reviews & Study Aids

A 400

B. Reactive lymph nodes.

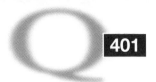

Q 401

This waveform was obtained
from which abdominal vessel?

a. renal vein

b. inferior vena cava

c. hepatic vein

d. inferior mesenteric artery

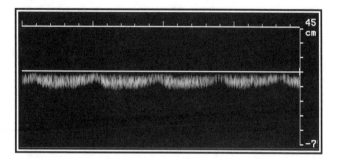

A 401

A. Renal vein.

The inferior vena cava and hepatic veins demonstrate highly pulsatile waveforms. The renal vein waveform shows respiratory phasicity but minimal pulsatility.

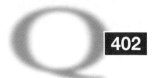

402

This sagittal image was obtained in the popliteal fossa in a patient with blue toe syndrome. What are the ultrasound findings?

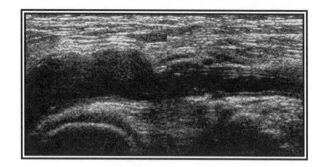

a. popliteal cyst

b. acute DVT popliteal vein

c. popliteal artery aneurysm

d. reactive lymph nodes

402

C. Popliteal artery aneurysm.

Q 403

This is a transverse image from the mid calf. Name the bones labeled A and B.

a. _____

b. _____

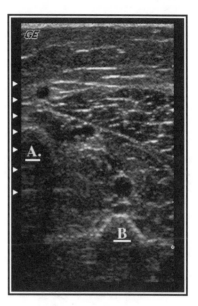

DAVIES
Registry Reviews & Study Aids

A **403**

A. Tibia.

B. Fibula.

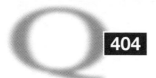

404

This transverse image was obtained in the upper arm. The brachial artery is seen with a brachial vein on each side. The small arrows are pointing to what vessel?

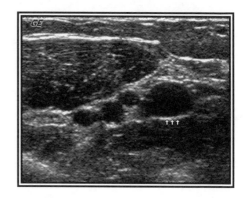

a. accessory brachial vein

b. cephalic vein

c. axillary vein

d. basilic vein

A 404

D. Basilic vein.

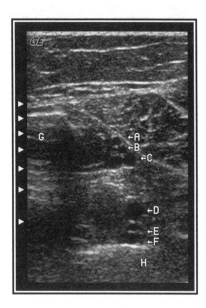

Q 405

This B-mode image was obtained in the upper calf. Name the vessels labeled A–F.

a. _____

b. _____

c. _____

d. _____

e. _____

f. _____

DAVIES
Registry Reviews & Study Aids

A 405

A. Posterior tibial vein.

B. Posterior tibial artery.

C. Posterior tibial vein.

D. Peroneal vein.

E. Peroneal artery.

F. Peroneal vein.

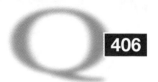

406

This waveform was obtained from the left vertebral artery. From this waveform, it can be determined that there is a stenosis in what vessel?

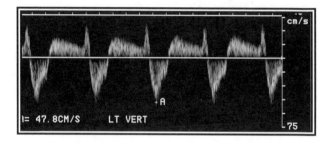

a. innominate artery

b. distal left vertebral

c. proximal left subclavian artery

d. distal left subclavian artery

A **406**

C. Proximal left subclavian artery.

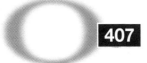

407

This is a transverse image of the left common carotid artery. Which statement below correctly describes this image?

a. smooth homogeneous plaque

b. ulcerated plaque

c. heterogeneous plaque with questionable intraplaque hemorrhage

d. homogeneous plaque with calcification

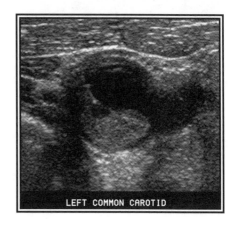

LEFT COMMON CAROTID

407

C. Heterogeneous plaque with questionable intraplaque hemorrhage.

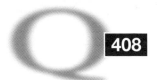

408

This waveform was obtained from
a fasting patient. Which vessel
below is the most likely source for
this Doppler trace?

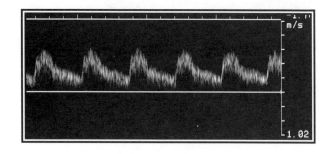

a. superior mesenteric artery

b. inferior mesenteric artery

c. celiac trunk

d. infrarenal abdominal aorta

A 408

C. Celiac trunk.

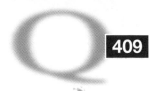

409

This Doppler waveform was obtained in a posterior tibial artery by sweeping the Doppler sample volume from <u>above</u> (proximal to) a graft anastomosis to <u>below</u> (distal to) the graft anastomosis. There is retrograde flow <u>above</u> the bypass graft anastomotic site. What is suggested by this finding?

a. arteriovenous fistula proximal to the graft anastomosis

b. normal back-flow up the native artery

c. stenosis in the distal native artery

d. stenosis in the graft

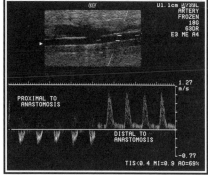

VIII. Image Gallery / Image-Based Cases and Questions

A 409

B. Normal back-flow up the native artery.

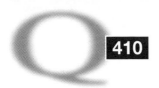

This Doppler waveform was obtained in a normal internal carotid artery. Which of the following could explain the loss of the spectral window?

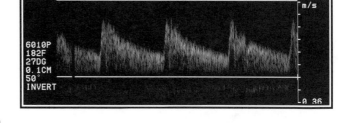

a. sample volume not centered in the artery

b. sample volume size too small

c. pulse repetition frequency too low

d. sweep speed set too low

A. Sample volume not centered in the artery.

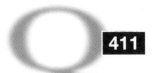

Q 411

This sagittal image was taken from the mid calf. The vein seen in this image emptied into a posterior tibial vein. What vein is being imaged?

a. gastrocnemius vein

b. sural vein

c. greater saphenous vein

d. soleal vein

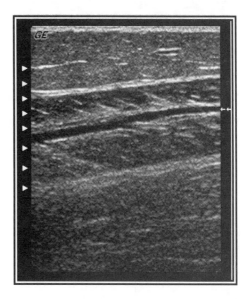

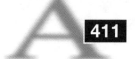

D. Soleal vein.

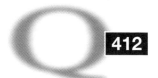

412

This sagittal B-mode image was taken with the probe positioned on the medial aspect of the mid calf. What pair of veins is being demonstrated?

a. posterior tibial veins

b. peroneal veins

c. lesser saphenous veins

d. soleal veins

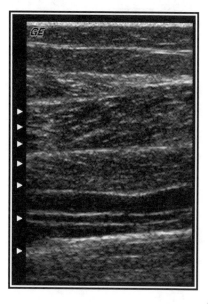

824

B. Peroneal veins.

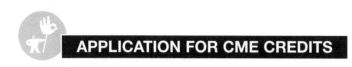

APPLICATION FOR CME CREDITS

**ScoreCards™
for Vascular Technology**

This continuing medical educational (CME) activity is approved for 7.5 hours of credit by the Society of Diagnostic Medical Sonographers. This credit may be applied as follows:

- Sonographers and technologists may apply these hours toward the CME requirements of the ARDMS, ARRT, and/or CCI, as well as to the CME requirements of ICAVL for technologists and sonographers in facilities accredited by that organization.

- Physicians may apply a certain maximum number of SDMS-approved credit hours toward the CME requirements of the ICAVL for accreditation of diagnostic facilities. (Be sure to confirm current requirements with the pertinent organizations.) Physicians who are registered sonographers or technologists may apply all of these hours toward the CME requirements of the ARDMS, ARRT, and/or CCI. SDMS-approved credit is not applicable toward the AMA Physician's Recognition Award.

If you have any questions whatsoever about CME requirements that affect you, please contact the responsible organization directly for current information. CME requirements can and sometimes do change.

DAVIES
Registry Reviews & Study Aids

NOTE

The original purchaser of this CME activity is entitled to submit this CME application for an administrative fee of $26.50. Please enclose a check payable to Davies Publishing Inc. with your application. Others may also submit applications for CME credits by completing the activity as explained above and enclosing an administrative fee of $36.50. The CME administrative fee helps to defray the cost of processing, evaluating, and maintaining a record of your application and the credit you earn. Fees may change without notice. For the current fee, call us at 626.792.3046, e-mail us at **daviescorp@aol.com,** or write to us at the aforementioned address. We will be happy to help!

Objectives of this Activity

Upon completion of this educational activity, you will be able to:

1 Identify the gross anatomy of the central and peripheral arterial and venous systems.

2 Describe the physiology and fluid dynamics of the central and peripheral circulation.

3 Describe how, when, and why imaging and nonimaging techniques are applied to the noninvasive diagnosis of vascular disease.

4 Describe the invasive tests and therapeutic interventions used in vascular disease.

5 List the diagnostic criteria for both imaging and nonimaging tests used in the noninvasive diagnosis of vascular disease.

6 Apply statistical techniques to the analysis of the sensitivity, specificity, accuracy, and negative and positive predictive values of a diagnostic test.

How to Obtain CME Credit

To apply for credit, please do all of the following:

1 Read and study the book and complete the interactive exercises it contains.

2 Photocopy and complete the following evaluation questionnaire (you grade us!) and CME quiz.

3 Return the completed forms together with payment of the administrative and processing fee (see Note above) to the following address:

CME Coordinator
Davies Publishing, Inc.
32 South Raymond Avenue, Suite 4
Pasadena, California 91105-1935

Please allow 15 working days for processing. Questions? Please call us at 626-792-3046.

4 If more than one person will be applying for credit, be sure to photocopy the applicant information, evaluation form, and CME quiz so that you always have the original on hand for use.

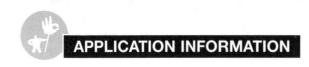

APPLICATION INFORMATION

Name   SSN

Your degrees and credentials

Street address

City/State/Zip

Telephone   Fax   eMail

ARDMS Registration #   ARRT Registration #   SDMS Member #

Signature and date certifying your completion of the activity

Evaluation—You Grade Us!

Please let us know what you think of the *ScoreCards* study system. Participating in this quality survey is a requirement for CME applicants, and it benefits future readers by ensuring that current readers are satisfied and, if not, that their comments and opinions are heard and taken into account.

1 Why did you purchase *ScoreCards*? (Circle your primary reason.)

Registry review   Course text   Clinical reference   CME activity

2 Have you used *ScoreCards* for other reasons, too? (Circle all that apply.)

Registry review   Course text   Clinical reference   CME activity

3 To what extent did *ScoreCards* meet its stated objectives and your needs? (Circle one.)

Greatly   Moderately   Minimally   Insignificantly

4 The content of *ScoreCards* was (circle one):

Just right   Too basic   Too advanced

5 The quality of the questions, explanations, illustrations, and case examples was mainly (circle one):

Excellent   Good   Fair   Poor

6 The manner in which *ScoreCards* presents the material is mainly (circle one):

Excellent   Good   Fair   Poor

7 If you used *ScoreCards* to prepare for the registry exam, did you also use other materials or take any exam-preparation courses?

No   Yes   (please specify what materials and courses)

_____

_____

8 If you used *ScoreCards* for a course, please name the course, the instructor's name, the name of the school or program, and any other textbooks you may have used:

Course/Instructor/School or program _____

_____

Other textbooks _____

9 What did you like best about *ScoreCards*?

_____

_____

_____

10 What did you like least about *ScoreCards*?

_____

_____

_____

11 If you used *ScoreCards* to prepare for your registry exam in vascular technology,
    did you pass?

   Yes   No   Haven't yet taken it

12 May we quote any of your comments in our catalogs or promotional material?

   Yes   No   Further comment

_____

_____

_____

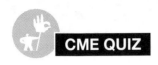

CME QUIZ

Please answer the following questions after you have completed the CME activity. There is one best answer for each question. Circle it.

1. What is the most common anatomic variation of the renal arteries?
   a. retroaortic renal artery
   b. multiple renal arteries
   c. congenital absence of one main renal artery
   d. anterocaval course of right renal artery

2. Which of the following vessels courses along the medial aspect of the psoas muscle?
   a. internal iliac artery
   b. external iliac artery
   c. femoral artery
   d. inferior mesenteric artery

3. The first branch of the external carotid artery is usually the:
   a. facial artery
   b. superficial temporal artery
   c. internal maxillary artery
   d. superior thyroid artery

5. Which vein in the antecubital fossa connects the cephalic and basilic veins?
    a. axillary vein
    b. median cubital vein
    c. cephalic vein
    d. basilic vein

6. Which statement is NOT true regarding the soleal veins?
    a. They empty into the posterior tibial or peroneal veins.
    b. They are found deep in the calf muscle.
    c. They connect with the superficial venous system.
    d. They do not contain valves.

7. Regarding the inferior vena cava, all of the statements below are true EXCEPT:
    a. The inferior vena cava drains into the left atrium of the heart.
    b. The inferior vena cava is formed by the confluence of the common iliac veins.
    c. The inferior vena cava has no valves below the level of its insertion into the heart.
    d. The inferior vena cava courses to the right of the abdominal aorta.

8. The major function of the vasa vasorum is to:
    a. regulate vasodilatation of the arterioles
    b. provide nourishment to the tunica adventitia
    c. provide the major communication in arteriovenous fistulas
    d. provide autoregulation of blood flow to the brain

9. The number of true positives divided by the number of true positives + false positives describes which of the following?
    a. sensitivity
    b. specificity
    c. accuracy
    d. positive predictive value

10. A percentage diameter reduction of 50% in a symmetric narrowing of the carotid artery most closely corresponds to what percentage area reduction?
    a. 35%
    b. 50%
    c. 75%
    d. 90%

11. Arteriovenous fistula is a complication that most commonly occurs with:
    a. reversed vein bypass grafts
    b. in situ grafts
    c. atherectomy
    d. angioplasty

12. A technique in which atherosclerotic plaque is mechanically removed by cutting or pulverizing it and then extracted by suction or downstream embolization is termed:
    a. atherectomy
    b. thrombectomy
    c. angioplasty
    d. endarterectomy

13. What severe symptom of decreased blood perfusion is aggravated by elevation, relieved by dependency, and often occurs when the patient goes to bed at night?
    a. claudication
    b. cyanosis
    c. rest pain
    d. postprandial pain

14. A nonatherosclerotic, noninflammatory, occlusive, and aneurysmal disorder that primarily affects women and is referred to as a "string of beads" is:
    a. Takayasu's disease
    b. mycotic aneurysm
    c. polyarteritis nodosa
    d. fibromuscular dysplasia

15. The most serious risk from femoropopliteal aneurysms is:
    a. rupture
    b. embolization
    c. fistula
    d. infection

16. A patient presents to the vascular lab with an abdominal bruit, weight loss, and postprandial pain. Obstruction of which vessel is most likely responsible for these symptoms?
    a. renal arteries
    b. portal vein
    c. superior mesenteric artery
    d. splenic vein

17. Palpation of a pulse found in the groove behind the medial malleolus of the ankle corresponds to the:
    a. posterior tibial artery
    b. anterior tibial artery
    c. peroneal artery
    d. plantar artery

18. An acceleration time of less than 133 msec obtained in the femoral artery suggests:
    a. proximal iliac artery stenosis
    b. distal femoral artery occlusion
    c. pseudoaneurysm of the femoral artery
    d. the absence of significant iliac artery disease

19. Reactive hyperemia testing is:
    a. an alternative method to treadmill exercise testing for stressing the peripheral arterial circulation
    b. a method to evaluate the flow patterns within veins
    c. a method utilized in the measurement of limb volume changes
    d. a method to rule out thoracic outlet syndrome

20. What measurement helps in differentiation of inflow versus outflow disease by measuring the time between the onset of systole to the maximum systolic peak?
    a. resistive index
    b. acceleration time
    c. volume flow
    d. A/B ratio

21. Following cessation of exercise in a normal individual, how long does it take for lower extremity blood flow to return to resting values?
    a. 1–5 minutes
    b. 5–10 minutes
    c. 10–15 minutes
    d. as long as 30 minutes

22. Which ABI is indicative of rest pain?
    a. > 1.0
    b. 0.9–1.0
    c. 0.5–0.9
    d. < 0.5

23. Arteriography is contraindicated in a patient with which condition?
    a. diabetic
    b. renal failure
    c. malignancy
    d. vascular disease

24. The biggest contributing risk factor for stroke is:
    a. hypertension
    b. hypercholesterolemia
    c. sedentary life style
    d. alcohol abuse

25. An abnormal sound heard on auscultation caused by flow turbulence is a:
    a. Bernoulli
    b. bruit
    c. Poiseuille
    d. thrill

26. The term *spectral broadening* describes:
    a. the length of the cardiac cycle
    b. a wide range of frequency shifts reflected back to the transducer
    c. a wide bandwidth continuous-wave Doppler
    d. reversed flow at any point during the cardiac cycle

27. The point at which aliasing occurs is known as the:
    a. Nyquist limit
    b. Poiseuille's point
    c. Bernoulli's equation
    d. Reynolds number

28. In transcranial Doppler, with the probe placed over the right temporal bone, flow in the right middle cerebral artery will be:
    a. oriented away from the probe
    b. oriented toward the probe
    c. oriented at 90° to the probe
    d. the right middle cerebral artery cannot be seen from this window

29. The presence of a mosaic pattern in the color Doppler image of the internal carotid artery most likely indicates:
    a. slow flow proximal to an occlusion
    b. the presence of poststenotic turbulence
    c. reversed flow in the vertebral artery
    d. improper color setup with the pulse repetition frequency set too high

30. Overestimation of the degree of stenosis in the internal carotid artery may be due to all of the following EXCEPT:
    a. increased velocities contralateral to an occlusion
    b. overestimation of the angle of incidence
    c. improper location of the sample volume proximal to the stenosis
    d. vessel tortuosity

31. Which of the following cannot be determined from an arteriogram?
    a. percent diameter stenosis
    b. reversed flow in the vertebral
    c. arterial dissection
    d. flow turbulence

32. Elevated peripheral venous pressure results in:
    a. edema
    b. decreased arterial resistance
    c. lymphangitis
    d. dependent rubor

33. Homan's sign is:
    a. a highly specific sign for lower extremity venous thrombosis
    b. a highly specific sign for upper extremity venous thrombosis
    c. calf discomfort on passive dorsiflexion
    d. numbness of the digits with hyperextension of an extremity

34. In the lower extremity, maximum flow return in the venous system is present with:
    a. inspiration
    b. expiration
    c. valsalva maneuver
    d. release of distal compression

35. Which of the following describes normal flow in the portal vein?
    a. hepatopetal
    b. hepatofugal
    c. triphasic
    d. bidirectional

36. With duplex sonography, the main purpose of probe compression is to:
    a. rule out incompetent valves
    b. rule out the presence of thrombus
    c. differentiate between superficial and deep veins
    d. differentiate between veins and arteries

37. Which is an advantage of color Doppler imaging over B-mode imaging alone in evaluation of the venous system?
    a. recanalized thrombi are more readily apparent
    b. partially occluding thrombi are better detected
    c. venous collaterals are more readily visualized
    d. all of the above

38. During the Valsalva maneuver, what happens to pressure in the abdomen and thorax?
    a. intrathoracic pressure increases, abdominal pressure increases
    b. intrathoracic pressure decreases, abdominal pressure decreases
    c. intrathoracic pressure increases, abdominal pressure decreases
    d. intrathoracic pressure decreases, abdominal pressure increases

39. In contrast venography, which finding would indicate the presence of a thrombus?
    a. contrast extravasation
    b. filling defect
    c. increase in opacity
    d. none of the above

40. Symptoms associated with thoracic outlet syndrome include all of the following EXCEPT:
    a. increased blood pressure on the affected side
    b. numbness or tingling of the arm
    c. aching of shoulder and forearm
    d. increased discomfort with upward arm positions

41. Blue toe syndrome is caused by:
    a. venous thrombosis of the pedal veins
    b. hyperemic flow from arteriovenous fistulas
    c. congenital absence of the dorsalis pedis artery
    d. embolization from proximal arteries

42. Which is a complication of dialysis access grafts?
    a. arterial steal
    b. aneurysm
    c. venous stenosis
    d. all of the above

43. The tendency of objects to maintain their status quo is called:
    a. kinetic energy
    b. potential energy
    c. inertia
    d. hydrostatic pressure

44. The term *phasicity,* in reference to the venous system, refers to:
    a. the influence of the cardiac cycle on venous flow
    b. the rate at which the valves open and close
    c. the ebb and flow in the veins that occurs in response to respiration
    d. the effect of intrinsic and extrinsic pressure on venous wall stiffness

45. Which of the following does NOT occur as a result of trauma?
    a. arteriovenous malformation
    b. arteriovenous fistula
    c. pseudoaneurysm
    d. dissection

NOTES